THE

HUNTER/FARMER

DIET SOLUTION

THE

HUNTER/FARMER
DIET SOLUTION

DO YOU HAVE THE METABOLISM OF A HUNTER
OR A FARMER? FIND OUT . . . AND ACHIEVE
YOUR HEALTH AND WEIGHT-LOSS GOALS!

MARK LIPONIS, M.D.

HAY HOUSE, INC.
Carlsbad, California • New York City
London • Sydney • Johannesburg
Vancouver • Hong Kong • New Delhi

Published and distributed in the United States by: Hay House, Inc.: www.hayhouse .com® • *Published and distributed in Australia by:* Hay House Australia Pty. Ltd.: www.hayhouse.com.au • *Published and distributed in the United Kingdom by:* Hay House UK, Ltd.: www.hayhouse.co.uk • *Published and distributed in the Republic of South Africa by:* Hay House SA (Pty), Ltd.: www.hayhouse.co.za • *Distributed in Canada by:* Raincoast: www.raincoast.com • *Published in India by:* Hay House Publishers India: www.hayhouse.co.in

Cover design: theBookDesigners • *Interior design:* Pamela Homan

Library of Congress Cataloging-in-Publication Data

Liponis, Mark.
    The Hunter/Farmer diet solution : do you have the metabolism of a Hunter or a Farmer? find out-- and achieve your health and weight-loss goals / Mark Liponis.
        p. cm.
    ISBN 978-1-4019-3553-5 (hardback)
1. Reducing diets. 2. Weight loss. 3. Metabolism--Regulation. 4. Self-care, Health.
I. Title.
    RM222.2.L5347 2012
    613.2'5--dc23
                                    2011047497

Hardcover ISBN: 978-1-4019-3553-5
Digital ISBN: 978-1-4019-3555-9

15 14 13 12   4 3 2 1
1st edition, April 2012

Printed in the United States of America

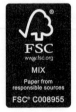

For my dad, Charlie Liponis,
an amazing man and towering role model
who always struggled with his weight,
God bless him.

CONTENTS

INTRODUCTION

We don't really need another diet. We need a solution.

We have to understand how to eat in a way that's right for us, a way that satisfies our cravings and helps us achieve and maintain a healthy weight. America is in the midst of a growing obesity epidemic. More than half of Americans are considered overweight, and more than a third obese.

Our national efforts to help restore the U.S. to a healthy weight have failed so far. Fad diets continue to flourish, and most people have experienced yo-yo dieting and weight swings. Losing weight is one of the top concerns of millions of Americans, and it's one of the most common reasons for patients coming to see me or spend time here at Canyon Ranch. We've gained tremendous experience in understanding what makes diets work when they do, and why they fail.

Still, it's sad to see the emotional impact of weight on so many wonderful men and women. Even very successful individuals often consider themselves failures if they're unable to control their weight. It affects their self-esteem and their perceived self-worth. For many it's as important as money or status.

In some ways it's not surprising that we've become overweight, because the ability to store energy (as fat) is a survival trait that's hardwired into our bodies. It makes sense to store extra energy as insurance against famine. But storing too much is also a problem, contributing to many of the health issues plaguing Americans such as diabetes, high blood pressure, heart disease, stroke, and cancer (in some cases), and more.

How has this normal survival tactic gone haywire, leading to obesity and poor health? Have we all just gotten lazy and sluggish and accustomed to overeating? No, not really. It's natural to gain weight over time when food is plentiful, but easy access to high-calorie, high-fat, and high-sugar foods has upset our traditional and ancestral ways of eating, effectively bypassing and undermining our body's natural ability to regulate appetite and weight. This easy access to the wrong kinds of food is the primary cause of rising obesity, with so many of us eating the wrong diet.

What we're beginning to understand is that the right diet is not just one diet, but it's *the right diet for the right person,* and there are different kinds of people when it comes to eating.

Eating right means eating right for *you,* and you may have already figured out what that means . . . or you might be interested in learning how to figure that out. You may find that some of your experiences and intuitions are valid, while some accepted "dogma" is just myth. I hope what you learn in these pages is helpful in reaching your weight and health goals.

🗡 🗡 🗡

CHAPTER ONE

MODERN-DAY HUNTERS AND FARMERS

Let me tell you about two people whom I've recently been working with. One of these is Beth, a 34-year-old part-time teacher from suburban Chicago. The other is Tom, a 42-year-old lawyer from Atlanta.

First Beth. Outwardly, she seems like someone who has everything going for her: she loves her job, she has a stable marriage and two healthy children, and she has so far been blessed with good health.

She does have one troubling issue: over the last ten years, Beth has gained 30 pounds. Once a woman who was proud of staying in good shape, her self-image had fallen to the point recently where she refused to shop for new clothes, devastated by having to look at herself in the mirror.

Beth found it easy to rationalize her weight gain over time, and she told herself the most important part of her life was taking care of her family. She felt happy in that regard; her children, a nine-year-old girl and a six-year-old boy, were involved in lots of kids' activities—dance, gymnastics, soccer, and music—and were healthy. Beth's husband, Greg, was even-keeled and solid, although he had his own business and worked very long hours, which meant that the couple spent less time together than Beth would have liked.

Over the years Beth's weight kept increasing; when she reached 160, she became highly agitated and envisioned herself ballooning to 200 pounds or more. She also worried—rightly—what effects her weight might be having on her health.

In a near panic attack, she broke down and sobbed to Greg, who tried to be reassuring but didn't know what to say; he suggested that if she felt this poorly, she might want to seek professional help. This only made Beth feel worse, because now she felt that she had failed as a mother and wife. Greg promised her this wasn't the case, and that all he cared about was her health and happiness.

He also suggested that maybe it was best for her to go on a getaway, maybe to a weight-loss spa. Greg's sister had gone to Canyon Ranch, and when he suggested it, Beth, after thanking Greg for his support, agreed.

At Canyon Ranch, when we first talked, Beth confessed that her secret fear was that her eating habits might be creating the possibility for a disease like diabetes or cancer. Her father had diabetes and had a heart stent, and his parents also had diabetes and heart problems, so there was a history of health issues to worry about.

She also explained that her weight had always been at 130 until the kids came along. Then things changed, and the pounds began to appear. When she reached 140, she would always panic and go on a diet, starving herself for days to lose five or six pounds until 135 became the new normal.

But, inevitably, the weight would creep back on until she passed the unthinkable 145. She would try another diet, repeating the same process: losing the weight, then gaining it again.

The more Beth and I talked, the more I learned about her past. She came from a close-knit family in which she was the middle of three children. A healthy baby, she weighed eight pounds at birth and never suffered from any serious illnesses. Growing up she was solid and athletic and liked playing sports, especially soccer. She did well in school and studied languages in college, eventually earning her teaching degree. She enjoyed her job at a local magnet school teaching Spanish.

Beth was a handsome woman with thick dark hair, big eyes, and soft features. She looked younger than her 34 years. And it was hard to see all those extra pounds at first glance. From the waist up, her figure didn't appear obese, and while her arms weren't thin, she appeared normally proportioned. Beth had gained mainly below the waist, around her hips, thighs, and buttocks. As a result, she had preserved her hourglass figure, but expanded particularly on the bottom. She also complained about the unsightly cellulite that had accumulated on her thighs and said she would love nothing more than to get rid of it.

Beth and I spoke at length about her diet. She liked a variety of foods, some of which were healthy. She often made chicken dishes, cooked up some meat a couple of times a week, and prepared fish every other week (but usually fried). She liked veggies and fruits but also cheese and butter. She drank too many diet sodas and had a hard time resisting potato chips and French fries, but that didn't happen too often. She refused to give up her double mocha latte in the morning, and she'd sometimes feel the need for a biscotti or bran muffin along with that.

On days that she worked, she usually brought lunch in with her, generally leftovers from last night's dinner or a sandwich or pasta salad, for example. She kept a couple bars of dark chocolate in her desk and had three or four squares at the end of the day before heading home. She cooked dinner on most nights and was diligent about making her family a healthy meal.

Twice a week they might order in—pizza or Chinese food—and she and Greg would go out for dinner and a movie once every week or two.

Beth brought in a copy of her most recent blood tests. Her cholesterol level was 240, and her doctor had told her that if she couldn't bring it down with diet, she might have to go on medication. The good news was that she did have a fairly high level of the "good" cholesterol known as HDL (high-density lipoprotein), which was at 65. But Beth's "bad" cholesterol level, or LDL, was also high at 160. Her doctor had not given her much advice on how to lower it but suggested that she could see a nutritionist, which she planned to pursue during her visit to Canyon Ranch.

I asked Beth what kind of success she'd had with losing weight in the past, and she told me that she had tried a number of different diets. And she'd had some small, temporary successes: She had lost six pounds with Weight Watchers but wasn't able to keep it up. She tried the Atkins diet and lost seven pounds but painfully and fairly quickly gained back ten when she stopped it.

I asked her why she stopped and she explained that she just didn't feel well on it—kind of queasy—and she also felt guilty about eating all that meat and cheese. She was worried what that might be doing to her cholesterol level and imagined her arteries clogging up as she lost weight. And within three weeks of stopping the Atkins diet, she was shocked to have gained ten pounds back. Beth panicked and went on a medical smoothie diet, eating only powdered meals mixed up in a blender for two weeks. After losing just three pounds, she gave up completely, never wanting another smoothie again.

Beth now hated even the idea of dieting; it made her feel deprived—and hungry. She said her friends and family had learned not to joke around with her when she was hungry because she lost her sense of humor. She also lost her ability to make a decision, and described how she couldn't buy a pair of shoes or grade students' papers if her blood sugar was low. That was when she was most likely to reach for a candy bar or some gummy bears to help keep her going.

Keeping hunger at bay was sometimes hard for Beth and she often found herself running out of energy, feeling exhausted and starving, especially come late afternoon.

Beth's story wasn't that unusual, because so many people struggle with their weight and don't always understand why. I then explained the concept of the Hunter/Farmer Diet to Beth. In terms of dietary needs, there are two basic kinds of people, and they need two different diets. There are the Farmers, who need a low-fat, grain-based diet. And there are Hunters, who need a low-carb diet based on protein and veggies.

❧ ❧ ❧

Beth was a typical Farmer, which was apparent from her body shape and blood results. Beth had big hips and thighs and a narrow waist. Her blood results also showed the typical Farmer pattern, with low glucose and triglycerides, and high cholesterol and HDL (more on this, later).

Farmers need to eat frequent small meals and snacks (while the Hunter is better suited to eating less often, maybe once or twice a day). Beth was typical of the Farmer type, getting hungry often and feeling weak and exhausted—symptoms of low blood sugar.

The Farmer is prone to low blood sugar, also known as glucose. When your glucose levels drop, you have less energy, you feel tired and weak, and you lose mental clarity; decision-making (among other things) becomes tough. That's because glucose is your main source of energy—it's your body's preferred fuel, and it's necessary for all bodily functions. Think of glucose as the gas that powers your muscles, heartbeat, breathing, and brain. If you run out of glucose, some functions will stop. Most important is brain function, which is entirely dependent on glucose—as glucose levels drop, you become irritable, then sluggish, and eventually unconscious.

Thankfully, your blood glucose level is normally maintained in a fairly precise range through the actions of the hormone insulin. Insulin is the lead actor on the stage of blood-sugar control, even though there are several supporting actors and actresses.

Your pancreas releases insulin after you eat, and that helps cells receive the glucose from your meal. Insulin is the key that opens a channel in your muscle and liver and other cells that allows them to soak in glucose like a sponge. Your cells need the glucose to make energy. If insulin isn't working, or if your blood sugar is low, the result is fatigue.

Farmers are prone to low blood sugar because they are particularly sensitive to the effects of the hormone insulin. Just a little insulin goes a long way for Farmers—the Farmers' cells soak up more glucose with even less insulin. Their cells have more glucose channels, and the Farmers' muscle and liver cells are more efficient at absorbing and storing glucose.

This sensitivity to insulin also produces several other Farmer features, including body shape and metabolism. We'll talk much more about all the Farmer features shortly.

The important point is that Farmers are prone to low blood sugar. Because of this tendency, the Farmer thrives on eating a diet that helps maintain blood sugar. The best foods for doing so are grains, such as wheat, oats, corn, rice, barley, quinoa, rye, spelt, and so on. (Grains are an excellent source of glucose, which is released from the digestion of carbohydrates in them.)

As Beth and I spoke, I also explained that the Farmer diet is a low-fat diet. By eating less fat, Beth would consume fewer calories and her hunger would be satisfied by small, frequent snacks. In addition, less fat would help keep her cholesterol and LDL down.

Beth's reaction was joyful—she loved carbs and said they always made her feel good. And she didn't think cutting out the fat would be that difficult. Sure, she'd miss the fries and chips, but she was already thinking of healthier alternatives.

Beth could remember times when she'd splurged on fatty foods and how that had seemed to pack on weight more than anything. She thought she could blame specific bulges on her hips and thighs to splurges on fried foods and ice cream.

I could tell by the look on her face that she was having an "Aha!" moment. She was already making the changes in her mind: baked potato instead of fries; broiled chicken and fish instead of fried; and lots of snacks during the day of granola, berries, and nonfat yogurt.

Beth left my office with hope. Her next stop was to sit with our nutritionist to learn how to eat for her type. When Beth departed the Ranch, she was empowered and rejuvenated, with a new enthusiasm and a realistic program. We then made a plan for her to return in three months to check in on her progress.

The three-month report was excellent: Beth had lost ten pounds and two inches off her hips! Her appetite was satisfied, and she had steady energy levels. She didn't feel deprived and knew she could stay with the diet. As a bonus, her cholesterol had dropped almost 40 points!

The Farmer diet worked fantastically for Beth. She learned to keep her hunger under control by eating small amounts of carbs often. She consumed fewer calories because she had cut her fat intake (and fat has more than double the calories of carbs, ounce for ounce), so she was able to eat more food and still be eating fewer calories. Beth was also satisfied because she was eating foods she really liked and didn't feel deprived. She felt like she could keep eating that way forever.

※ ※ ※

Right around the same time I met Beth, I was also introduced to Tom. Tom had come to Canyon Ranch from Atlanta, Georgia, with his wife, Sue, who had been to the Ranch once before and had attended several lectures on nutrition and weight loss. She thought about how much

Tom could benefit from a few days here and made herself a promise to bring him.

Four weeks later, Tom was sitting in my office telling me about himself.

Tom was a large man who spoke with a nice Southern drawl as he described his successful law practice. The firm had expanded in a recent merger and Tom became a partner, which meant working even more than usual. Tom had been putting in 70-hour workweeks, not counting numerous business dinners and other evening events. He was a member at the local country club, but had only played three rounds of golf all summer—the sum total of his recent exercise.

What had brought Tom to my office was the issue of weight: in the past two years, he had gained 40 pounds. He was tired and sleep deprived. At 42, he confessed to already feeling middle-aged.

So far Tom had avoided any health crisis—he and Sue considered this visit preemptive. But he knew his current lifestyle was not sustainable. He had to make some changes, and he knew that getting his weight and eating under control were the most important.

The bad news was that Tom's diet was a disaster. He'd pump sugar and caffeine into his system in the morning to get going—at least three mugs of high-test coffee with cream and sugar accompanied by a honey-dipped cruller or chocolate doughnut. On weekends he usually ate big bowls of cereal with fruit. During the week, Tom almost always worked through lunch, but there were occasional business luncheons with the usual steak and fries fare and a drink or two.

Afternoons Tom would meet with clients and work late, not leaving the office until 7:30 or 8. In the meantime, he'd drink a couple sodas and down a bag of cookies or a chocolate bar.

Most evenings meant gatherings, dinners, or events; the other nights he'd be home and eat a decent meal, cooked by Sue. His favorite meal was pasta, but he also enjoyed a steak at least twice a week. He could never resist a warm bun or a piece or two of bread.

At functions and dinners, Tom would often drink three or four glasses of wine; at home the couple usually didn't drink unless guests were coming over; he didn't smoke except perhaps a cigar or two when he was playing golf, which was happening less and less.

Tom was sincere in his desire to get a grip on his weight and his health. He worried about his heart, especially since one of his firm's partners, just two years older, had recently had a heart attack and got a heart stent. Tom had passed a stress test a few years earlier for a life-insurance physical, but he'd gained a lot of weight since then.

He was also worried about his blood pressure; he'd never had a high reading until this past year when an insurance health screen found his blood pressure to be high.

Tom was aware of the link between belly fat, heart disease, and high blood pressure; and looking at himself he recognized the typical apple shape: almost all of the weight he had gained had come in his belly, chest, and face; almost none in his legs or arms. He was still able to use the same belt for the past few years, but his shirt and jacket size had grown three times.

Tom also knew about the link between stress and weight, and that's where he placed the blame for his decline. He hoped that would change now that the business merger was complete. It was a good time for Tom to set some new goals and priorities; Sue's instincts were good ones and the timing was perfect.

Tom had a complete checkup including a physical, stress test, and blood work. His body fat was a high 40 percent, and most of that was in his belly—his legs and arms were only 22 percent fat by comparison. His blood pressure was mildly elevated at 140/92. The top number signifies the pressure in the arteries while the heart is squeezing, and the bottom number measures the pressure when the heart is relaxed and filling. Normal blood pressure is 120/80 or below. With exercise, Tom's blood pressure went up even higher to 220/100 and he looked red-faced, huffing and puffing on the treadmill during his stress test. Analyzing Tom's cardiac EKG, it looked as though there could be small, partial blockages.

Another scare came from the blood results, which showed a number of problems. Tom's blood sugar (glucose) was elevated on the borderline of diabetes. His cholesterol was high, and the level of HDL or "good" cholesterol was too low. Those all increased his risk of heart attack. Also, his liver tests showed a "fatty liver," which is sort of like a foie gras liver in a human. (Foie gras is a French delicacy—the fatty liver of a goose—caused by force-feeding the geese).

All this added up to bad news, but Tom couldn't deny the results from the tests, which showed him heading rapidly toward diabetes and heart and liver problems. The good news was that Tom made a commitment to change—he just needed to know what to change and how.

I asked Tom if he'd ever had any success losing weight before. He had tried dieting several times over the past few years, but the results hadn't been good. He'd begun working with a nutritionist for a couple months who gave him more structured meals and started off with a big breakfast every morning to curb his appetite during the day, but Tom found he was still eating a big dinner many nights. He sensed alcohol may have been contributing to his weight gain and tried cutting that out for a while and lost four pounds, but he quickly put the weight back on.

He also tried the South Beach Diet because everyone at work seemed to be on it; he lost about eight pounds the first few weeks, but then plateaued and didn't lose anything the next few weeks. At that point he lost interest and gave up, and the weight returned over the next couple months.

Tom thought some more incentive might help him, so he made a bet with one of his partners for $100 a pound for a month—each had to pay the other $100 for each pound they lost over a month's time. That ended up being a complete failure—neither of them believed the other would be successful, and in the end Tom ended up gaining three pounds that month while his partner stayed the same. Tom lost $300. That experience was difficult for Tom, because he really felt like a failure and wondered if he would ever be able to lose weight and keep it off.

It was especially frustrating because he felt so competent and successful in all of the other areas of his life, but an utter failure when it came to weight.

For a guy who was overweight, he didn't think that he ate that much. In fact, Tom explained that he wasn't even very hungry most of the time. He would wake up in the morning and just want his cup of coffee. On the way to work, he'd grab a second cup and that's when he'd have his cruller. He explained that it wasn't hunger that made him buy the cruller; it was more habit, and a kind of craving.

He often found himself craving some kind of "pick-me-up" more than food, so he was more inclined to have a cup of coffee, or a soda and some cookies. He felt he was just looking for an energy boost or a mood lift.

Tom also realized that eating sometimes sapped his energy level and interfered with his ability to focus and concentrate. He realized that if he had a business luncheon, he'd often experience a wave of fatigue afterward that might make him need to lie on the couch and take a 20-minute nap. This happened most often when he had pasta and bread.

It wasn't until the end of the day—once he had finished his work and started to unwind—that he started actually feeling hungry, and dinner was his biggest meal. In fact, between dinner and bedtime, Tom would eat or drink 80 percent of all of his calories for the day.

Tom was eager for help and ready to make the necessary changes.

The first step was to give Tom an understanding of how he should think about food. I explained that he was a typical example of a Hunter, which was evident by his body shape and blood-test results. Tom gained most of his weight in his belly, and his legs and butt stayed slim. His blood work showed the classic Hunter findings: high blood glucose and triglycerides, and low HDL cholesterol (more on this, later).

Hunters are good at being able to go for longer periods of time without eating. They experience less hunger and are more likely to "feast" than to "graze." Hunters crave sugar and carbohydrates, but get fatigued if they eat too much.

Hunters have more belly fat, so they develop the "apple shape" as they gain weight. Tom, typical of the Hunter type, had gained most of his extra fat in his belly and chest and very little in his hips/thighs and legs. He also fit the

Hunter type in terms of his craving of sugar and carbs, and his pattern of hunger, which was infrequent.

The reason why Tom struggled with his weight is that he had been eating the wrong diet. If he continued with his present habits, he would be diabetic, soon. Tom was getting too much sugar from sugar itself, as well as from simple carbohydrates, which are quickly converted in the body to sugar. The sugar in Tom's coffee, the crullers and cookies, the pasta dishes and bread, and alcohol were all adding to the problem.

I explained to Tom that a Hunter needs a Hunter diet, which is high in protein and avoids refined grains, simple sugars, and starches. It is a low-glycemic diet. The reason for calling it the Hunter diet is that it's similar to the diet of a typical hunter-gatherer—higher in meat, fish, and eggs, and lower in grains.

These words resonated with Tom and his life: the carb craving, the appetite pattern, and the huge belly that he had grown. He was ready and eager to start on his new eating plan; and to help him understand it even more, his next stop was with his nutritionist at Canyon Ranch.

In a couple sessions he was equipped with a new strategy and weekly meal plans and recipes. We agreed that, like Beth, he would see me in three months. When he did, he reported that he had lost almost 20 pounds and felt terrific. He was sleeping better, he had more energy, and his belly had shrunk considerably. We rechecked Tom's blood, and his blood sugar was down to almost normal at 101. His triglycerides had dropped 100 points from 240 down to 140, and his HDL level improved by 20 percent. That was great progress for only three months.

Tom was thrilled. He said he knew he could continue his new lifestyle and reach his goals. We decided to get together again in a few months, and by his next visit, Tom had plateaued at his goal and ideal weight. He laughed about how easy it seemed and how he wished he had known about the Hunter diet years earlier. He said that he knew he would never be overweight again, and he left Canyon Ranch feeling confident and successful.

✍ ✍ ✍

CHAPTER TWO

A LIFE OF DIETS

It's gratifying to see great results and happy patients like Beth and Tom. It's also great to see their health improve and know that they're feeling better. That's the best thing about healthy weight loss: people feel better, and they feel better about themselves; losing weight helps them become both healthier *and* happier. Getting people on the right diet and seeing them succeed makes all the work of becoming a doctor worthwhile.

I'm so fortunate to see this kind of success on a regular basis here at Canyon Ranch, where I work as the chief Corporate Medical Director. Canyon Ranch is the world's best health spa—one of the first and only health spas in the U.S. to combine a comprehensive medical checkup with a luxurious, healthy getaway vacation. The Canyon Ranch programs help people with any variety of health issues, but we're especially known for helping people lose weight.

Canyon Ranch started in 1979 as sort of a "fat farm" for the rich and famous. The approach to weight loss has evolved considerably over the past three decades, as we've learned from the experience of hundreds of thousands of guests who have visited over the years.

Back in the early days of Canyon Ranch, the weight-loss strategy was much different—it consisted of a spartan diet of 800 calories a day combined with hours of hiking and group aerobics classes. People would come for a week or two and expect to lose a pound a day, but invariably the weight would come back when they returned home to their regular lives and diets. They weren't able to sustain that kind of calorie restriction and heavy exercise.

Eventually we learned that people needed a strategy that they could actually continue to follow successfully after leaving the Ranch, one that was sustainable and sensible. We also learned that different people needed different diets, but more on that later.

Long before I had ever heard of Canyon Ranch, I had developed an understanding of the important link between weight and health. Like many young doctors, early in my career I was attracted to the more action-packed areas of medicine: critical and emergency care. Being something of an adrenaline junkie, I loved the excitement. There's also immediate gratification; when someone is seriously ill, per-haps having heart trouble or difficulty breathing, you can help save a life. That kind of intensity is exciting and often scary, but it's also rewarding. For the first few years of my career as a doctor, that excitement kept me going.

But as time went on, I realized that I was just giving people a temporary fix. I hadn't really provided a cure—I had helped them through one crisis. Once they recovered, they still had the same basic problems that put them there. They still had heart disease or diabetes or high blood pres-sure, and so on.

I also began learning that most of my patients' illnesses were preventable! For one, I noticed that weight was often a factor in those life-threatening catastrophes. The majority of my younger critically ill patients were overweight, and their weight was usually a primary factor in their illness: Their weight was leading them to diabetes, or their diets were raising their cholesterol or blood pressure. Obesity was putting excessive strain on their hearts and lungs and making it more difficult for them to breathe and for their hearts to supply their bodies with blood.

My own mood started to change. What was initially thrilling and gratifying—saving lives—did not feel as good when I started seeing the same patients I had saved get sicker and eventually die from the same problems that had made them ill to start with. My attitude was turning cynical. I sometimes wondered if my efforts were totally in vain, and even questioned if perhaps I was contributing to the problem rather than solving it: saving people so they could go and get sick, again. It didn't feel like saving a life; it started to feel like prolonging bad health. I craved a better, long-term, and more gratifying solution.

I also realized that being able to show patients how to lose weight would be the single most important thing I could do. Weight loss was a sustainable solution, because only by losing weight could many of my patients finally shake their diabetes, control their blood pressure, and actually prevent themselves from getting sick to start with.

But in those days, we knew almost nothing about weight loss. It didn't matter. I knew that was the right thing to do, so I opened my own weight-loss clinic in 1992 called Practical Weight Loss. I hired a fantastic nurse, Leslie, who embodied all of the best qualities of a nurse, mother, coach, and cheerleader. We signed up hundreds of people and our program was very successful.

Leslie met with all our patients every week, and would ask me to meet with anyone who was having a particularly difficult time. We also started a support group and had a daily morning walk that Leslie led. It was like a little Canyon Ranch right in Butte, Montana, where I was living at the time.

Back then we put everyone on a low-fat diet—the accepted wisdom of the moment. We taught our patients how to count fat grams and to avoid fat like the plague. We reasoned that fat had twice the calories of carbs, and after all, people were trying to lose fat, not muscle. So cutting out dietary fat seemed like the perfect strategy.

It worked pretty well. Most people were losing weight.

Then, after our program had been running about a year, Leslie came to me with a stack of charts of some our clients who were struggling. But Leslie had a puzzled look on her face that made me pause. Something was unusual about these people, she explained. They were following the program, they had cut out fat, and they were writing down everything they were eating; it all seemed right. I didn't think they were lying.

But they weren't losing weight. They were following the program and joining in with the exercise and support groups. They seemed to be doing what everyone else was doing—but they just weren't making any progress. What made Leslie really wonder about them was what was happening to their blood work.

In our program, we tracked everyone's blood results: blood sugar, cholesterol, triglycerides, and so forth. Something about these particular patients wasn't adding up. Despite them being on the program for at least three months, not only weren't they losing weight, but their blood results also seemed to be getting worse. Their blood sugar, cholesterol, and triglyceride levels were going up, not down like most of our clients. They simply were not responding to the program like the others.

That was the very first time I realized that a low-fat diet does *not* work for everyone.

In fact, I could see that some of my patients actually got worse on one. It would take me several more years to figure out why, and how to find out which diet was best for those patients. But for that I would have to wait for my own "Aha!" moment to come.

Two years later, my family's time in Montana was coming to an end. My wife, Siobhan, and I were feeling disconnected from our extended families. Three young kids made it tougher to travel and we found ourselves seeing our parents, grandparents, cousins, uncles, and aunts less and less often. So we decided it was time to move back East to be closer to our loved ones. We packed up the kids, dogs, cars, bikes, and skis and headed to Massachusetts.

As fate would have it, we settled in the town of Lenox, in the Berkshire Hills of western Massachusetts. It's an idyllic setting, a great place to raise children.

Siobhan, who is a pediatrician, and I both found jobs easily. We settled in, and I began working in emergency departments at local hospitals around the area. It was hard work, especially the frequent night shifts, and I started looking for something that would be a little less stressful. I also felt like I was back practicing "finger in the dike" catastrophic medicine and longed once again to get into a practice where I could really make a difference with prevention.

That's when I stumbled across Canyon Ranch. In 1994 we had just moved into a rental house in a nice neighborhood that happened to be right across the street from a long, winding, beautiful driveway that led to a mansion at the top of a hill. A discreet sign said "Canyon Ranch."

I knew very little about the place at that time, but I started asking people about it. Most told me it was a "fat farm for movie stars," and I imagined chaise lounges lined up with the likes of Roseanne Barr and Marlon Brando getting manicures and massages while they sipped diet drinks and ate cucumber slices and caviar. I wondered what kind of diets they used, and I imagined various fad diets and lots of pampering.

However, my imagination couldn't have been further from the truth, as I learned that most guests at Canyon Ranch weren't celebrities at all; and the program included a full menu of exercise classes, hiking, canoeing, tennis, yoga, and in-depth medical exams as much as it did pampering and beautifying.

Oddly, a position at the Ranch soon opened up, and after just a few weeks, it was clearly a perfect match. I learned that Canyon Ranch's weight-loss program also included a strong medical component, as well as nutrition, fitness, and behavioral counseling. Ranch guests were generally affluent, but also struggling with the same problems with weight that everyone else was dealing with. The only difference was that they could afford getting the best help.

They also had a lot of curiosity and wanted to be tested to learn more about their bodies and metabolism. It was from this kind of constant analyzing and discovering patterns in the test results that I learned how people's metabolisms differ and which diets work best for which people.

Now men and women come from around the world to go through the Canyon Ranch Weight-Loss Program. The program includes consultations with our physician, nutritionist, exercise physiologist, and behavioral specialist. Cooking classes, lectures, and fitness classes help our clients learn the right ways to cook, eat, and exercise. The food in the dining room is no longer spartan or bland; it's abundant and flavorful. The menus are labeled with nutritional facts so guests can make the best decisions for themselves. Fat and carb grams are highlighted, as well as protein and fiber.

The result is that people can learn about and eat the diet that's best for them while realizing there's an abundance of choices. Recognizing that different people need different diets and providing the opportunity for them to eat as they should has been a big part of the success of Canyon Ranch and our Weight-Loss Program.

The past two decades of helping people lose weight have given me invaluable insight in helping my patients choose the right diet. I've learned that it's much easier for individuals to lose weight when they're on the right diet, and much more difficult for them when it's wrong.

The key is knowing which diet is right for you. As with Beth and Tom, you have to know whether you are a Farmer or Hunter. (If you want to skip ahead and take the Hunter/Farmer Quiz to figure out which type you are, turn to page 49.)

Different Diets for Different People

Of course it makes sense that different people need different diets. People are different! It's pretty obvious. We come from different families and backgrounds, and we're all different sizes and shapes and have different genes.

Scientists, artists, yogis, and even psychologists have tried to categorize the different human types with a variety of classifications. Dr. William Sheldon was an American psychologist who described the three physical types, or "somatotypes," known as *endomorph, ectomorph,* and *mesomorph.* Dr. Sheldon proposed that each somatotype was also linked with specific and different personality traits. Endomorphs were rounded and thicker people and demonstrated personality traits of good humor and evenness of emotions. Ectomorphs, on the other hand, had thinner and more delicate builds and emotional traits typified by introversion, artistic tendencies, social anxiety, and inhibition. Mesomorphs were described as naturally muscular and fit people with broad shoulders and narrow hips; and their personality was described as bold, risk-taking, adventure-seeking, and extroverted.

The time-honored Eastern tradition of Ayurveda, an Indian system of health and well-being, also identifies three types of constitutions, or "doshas," called *kapha, pitta,* and *vata.* Each type or dosha is characterized by a physical appearance, or "prakrti," as well as a particular personality type.

Today's media is full of popular articles about body shape, most often compared to common fruits like apples and pears. Doctors have found particular shapes to carry common health risks—for example, those who are apple shaped are more prone to heart attacks and diabetes.

Even as far back as in ancient Greece, Plato described three different types of people in his book *The Republic,* and he related each personality type with unique physical and temperamental qualities, as well as political ones. Moreover, astrologers and modern philosophers have also described different "body types" that match astrological signs or personality traits and dispositions.

Suffice it to say that there has been ample historical exploration of whether different categories of body type exist and how they relate to other traits, whether they are personality, psychology, or political orientation.

What I find most interesting is that all of the attempts to categorize human beings start with the presumption that each of us has a type, and that type is innate. We were born with it. So whether we gain weight or lose it; or our appearance changes; or even if our mood, attitude, or behavior fluctuates, we still have a basic essence or constitution that stays the same throughout our lives.

Just losing weight or building muscle can't turn an "apple" shape into a "pear" shape. Nor can a kapha constitution become vata, or an ectomorph become an endomorph. But it's perfectly possible for an apple to be a healthy apple, or a pear a healthy pear. Keeping a healthy weight is one of the single most important ways of maintaining good health, no matter which is your body type. Becoming obese is unhealthy whether you're an apple or a pear.

But even if you do or have become obese, you still have a basic constitution that you inherited from your predecessors—your genes.

And your genes are crucial when it comes to your health, your weight, and the best diet for you. We are entering the age of *nutrigenomics*, where genetic tests can predict the best diet for you. The science is still new, but there have been some early and significant discoveries that can help us distinguish the Hunters from the Farmers.

※ ※ ※

Some very intriguing clues were uncovered recently as part of a head-to-head diet study called the "A to Z Weight

Loss Study." This pivotal work was the first to directly compare the results of four popular diets. The diets were the low-carb Atkins diet, the low-fat Ornish diet, the LEARN behavior-modification diet, and the Zone Diet (hence, *A to Z*). The diets represented a range of carbohydrate intake from the low-carb Atkins to the high-carb Ornish, with Zone and LEARN in between.

Over a 12-month period, the Atkins diet followers consumed 34 percent carbs, the Zone diet 45 percent carbs, LEARN diet 47 percent carbs, and Ornish diet 52 percent carbs as a percentage of energy intake. Conversely, Ornish was the lowest fat and Atkins the highest. Therefore, the Atkins diet is most like the Hunter diet, and Ornish is most like the Farmer diet, as you will soon see.

The results showed that on average the participants did lose weight on all four diets, and they were also able to keep the weight off, at least for a year if they continued their specific plan.

At baseline, patients averaged 187 pounds, and after a year of dieting, the average weight loss was about 6.1 pounds for all of the participants. As a group, those following the Atkins diet lost the most (averaging 10.3 pounds) compared with 3.5 pounds for Zone, 4.8 pounds for LEARN, and 5.7 pounds for Ornish.

To many, the cholesterol results were surprising. Atkins (lowest carb) followers had better HDL values (the "good" cholesterol) and improved triglycerides, while LDL at two months was better with the Ornish (low-fat) diet. In addition to weight loss, Atkins was also best at reducing blood pressure. Surprisingly, the lowest-carb/highest-fat diet (Atkins) produced the best outcomes for both weight loss and improvement in cardiovascular health.

The most striking finding of the study was the huge variation in the amount of weight gained or lost by different people on the same diets. Within each diet category, there were some who had lost 30 or 40 pounds while others gained 10 pounds—meaning that people on the same diet had a range of 40 or 50 pounds of weight change! That's at least four or five times the average difference between the four diets.

Some dieters did great on a low-carb diet (losing up to 30 or 40 pounds), while others gained 10 pounds. The same was true on the low-fat (Ornish) diet, even though the calorie intakes were roughly the same.

How can we explain why some people are better suited for a low-carb diet, while others a low-fat diet? Genetics may be the key. To try to sort this out, DNA samples were collected for 138 of the 311 participants of the "A to Z" study.

The analysis showed that those with a few genes that favored a low-carb diet lost two and a half times the amount of weight compared with those on the same diet without the "low-carb genes." The same was true for the people whose genes favored a low-fat diet; they lost significantly more weight on a low-fat diet as those without the predisposing genes.

In other words, matching the right diet with the right person produced more than double the weight loss on average, and genes could predict which people would do best on which diet. Genetic differences finally explained the successes and failures on the low-carb versus low-fat diets! Now we know for certain that some of us are genetically programmed for low-carb diets (Hunters) and others low-fat diets (Farmers).

To date, studies suggest that about 45 percent of Caucasians have the low-carb genotype, and roughly 39 percent have the low-fat genotype. Three genes, so far, have been identified as key metabolic factors—called BP2, ADRB2, and PPAR-gamma—and they help to control the body's use of carbs and fats. It's almost certain that more genes will be discovered as important or even more important in determining the connection between our genes and optimal diets.

The Evolution of Eating

Why did nature create two types of humans with different metabolisms and dietary needs? This was most likely a result of the evolution of eating: how our ancestors survived and found food. No one knows exactly what the earliest humans ate, but it seems they were mostly carnivores. Digs at ancient archaeological sites around the world have unearthed a variety of tools, weapons, cooking utensils, and fireplaces that hold small pieces of evidence and clues about the eating habits of the earliest humans.

Our species is thought to have existed for around 200,000 years, although recent discoveries of the remains of very ancient human teeth in the Middle East may stretch that time frame back as much as 400,000 years. Still, as of now, the oldest Homo sapiens remains (found in Ethiopia) date to around 195,000 years ago.

The site of human origins in Africa was in one of the lushest climates in the world at that time, home to abundant species of plants and animals. Humankind was a fairly latecomer into the world, one already populated with animals like giant warthogs, African wolves, buffalo, hippopotamuses, and antelope. Plant species were robust and plentiful. There were freshwater lakes and open grasslands.

The earliest humans survived by foraging for edible plants, roots, berries, and fruits while also hunting both small and large animals. They were fortunate to have arisen on a continent that had both a hospitable climate and an abundant supply of plant and animal foods available. In addition, Africa was home to several large-game species such as water buffalo and antelope, which provided excellent hunting for the earliest humans.

Spears and thrown projectiles have been found with remains throughout Africa and Europe. Butchered bones of large animals including deer and even elephants testify to humankind's hunting proclivities.

Neanderthals lived across central Europe and the Mediterranean for as much as 100,000 years until as recently as 30,000 years ago. It's debated whether or not Neanderthals were true humans, but we know they shared a common ancestor with us about 500,000 years ago. Archaeological sites show that the Neanderthal's diet was primarily carnivorous, though they also cooked vegetables.

Cro-Magnons succeeded Neanderthals across Europe and, like the Neanderthals, they were hunters, specializing in large game like mammoths, deer, and bears. This source of food was fairly plentiful at the time and provided a great source of protein and calories, as well as hides, claws, and horns. It's clear that our early ancestors were hunters, but they also knew how to forage for fruit, nuts, leaves, and roots. As far back as 164,000 years ago, humans were also eating shellfish, and by 90,000 years ago were fishing with tools. So fish became an early part of humans' diet.

It wasn't until the last 12,000 years that humans shifted over from hunting and gathering food to producing it. Cultivation, herding, and animal husbandry provided relatively recent additions to our food sources. By that time, human migration had spread our species around the globe. For instance, we had already expanded across Eurasia and the Far East, north to Siberia, and across the Bering Strait into the Americas. (Humans had already populated Asia, Indonesia, Australia, and New Zealand 20,000 years earlier.)

Cultivation of crops is believed to have begun in the Fertile Crescent in the Middle East (the Tigris-Euphrates River basin in and around present-day Iraq). Farming also appeared independently in China, Africa, the Americas, and New Guinea not long after the Middle East. It's not understood exactly why cultivation began, but what is known is that it fundamentally changed our eating by providing a steady source of grains.

The earliest crops cultivated were the wild grains of the land, which were then selected and eventually hybridized to bring out the most desirable traits. Over time almost every culture had acquired a preferred grain and became adept at farming it.

Wheat and rye were among the first to emerge, with archeological evidence pointing to Syria at around 13,000 years ago as the likely place and time of their initial cultivation. Barley production can be traced back to about 10,500 years ago in the Fertile Crescent. Evidence found in northern China shows that millet had been cultivated by the Cishan beginning around 10,000 years ago, and in southern and eastern China, there is evidence of the early cultivation of rice dating to around 7,000 to 10,000 B.C. Maize appears to have been first cultivated in present-day Mexico at around 9,000 years ago. Quinoa is a relative newcomer grain, with evidence of its cultivation dating back to about 3,500 years ago in the area of present-day Bolivia and Peru.

Not long after learning to cultivate grain, humans learned how to increase the yield of each planting, and also learned how to concentrate it and store it in the strongest possible form. Grains were turned into whiskey, sake, and beer; cane and beets into sugar.

By 7000 B.C., domestication of animals had occurred, with pigs and goats among the first.

To summarize, farming and cultivation of grains and other crops are quite a recent discovery in the long history of the human race, and one that occurred long after humans had migrated across the globe.

Farming allowed the human race to be able to develop to its amazing capacity, because it created the potential for new occupations. If you could buy your food or trade for it, then you could pursue another occupation that didn't require you to grow or hunt food. Farming fueled the Bronze Age and catapulted humans forward in their cultural and technological development. Farming also fed the first armies and fueled the creation of the world's first empires in Egypt and Sumeria.

Another effect of farming and abundance of food was an accelerated birth rate. Cultures that adopted farming techniques experienced rapid growth and an increased reproductive rate. The combination of a sedentary lifestyle and a plentiful food supply produced a bumper crop of babies—and big babies, at that.

Hunter-gatherer populations were nomadic, mobile peoples subjected to the stresses of climate change, availability of resources, shifting populations, and harsh weather. Babies placed added strain on a system with already limited resources, and thus those born to nomadic, hunter-gatherer families were fewer and smaller in size. Perhaps it's a natural protection; smaller babies are easier to carry when you're moving, and they eat less food. (As you'll soon see, lower birth weight is a significant trait of the Hunter type.)

Farming, on the other hand—which provided a stable, more sedentary lifestyle and ready access to calories—created a boom for bigger babies. Studies show that a baby's size is an important predictor of future body type, metabolism, and dietary needs, and can even help predict future health risks. Bigger babies have bigger appetites and need a steady source of food. It makes sense that Farmer families could feed bigger babies because of the surplus and abundance of food from farming.

Farming, which also fueled the growth and development of human communities, ultimately contributed to the obesity epidemic we're experiencing now. A sedentary lifestyle with ready access to high-calorie foods and concentrated calories (sugar and alcohol, for instance) proved a recipe for disaster, especially when brought to a predominantly meat-eating population of hunters and gatherers.

That disaster has reached epic proportions, with unprecedented rates of obesity and diabetes, to the point where almost one in two Americans is overweight, and one in three is obese. Currently, one in ten is diabetic, and the rate of diabetes is expected to continue to rise. Projections estimate that one in every three Americans will be diabetic by the year 2050! And it's not just a problem in the U.S.; there are many examples of growing obesity rates in other countries coinciding with growing economies.

In many parts of the world previously thought to be protected from "Western diseases," such as diabetes and heart disease, there are now growing epidemics of conditions associated with obesity. China, India, the Middle East,

Latin America, and the Caribbean are all experiencing a rise in cases of diabetes and heart disease. According to the World Health Organization, more than 60 percent of worldwide occurrences of coronary heart disease can now be found in developing countries. Farming has been the primary force in contributing to this growing epidemic.

So what are we to do? Do we go back to eating buffalo meat and living in tents, or can we learn to change our eating habits as we've learned our farming skills?

The answer is that some of us should still be eating the "original" human, or Hunter, diet, and others should be eating a more plant-based Farmer's diet.

✻ ✻ ✻

Take Lindsey, for example. A smart and successful lawyer, Lindsey worked almost constantly. Then, on her 50th birthday, she took her first break in a decade and visited Canyon Ranch. She wanted to relax and lose weight. Lindsey's nonstop lifestyle didn't lend itself to good health; her lack of exercise and poor eating habits had packed on the weight, and for the first time in her life, she was more than 200 pounds.

Lindsey knew this had to be affecting her health. To make matters worse, she was going through menopause and struggling with that, too. It's the kind of perfect storm that's common for many people who arrive at midlife only to realize they had better change something before it's too late.

When we met, I asked Lindsey for more details about her diet. She explained that she thought she might have a problem with sugar and that she was always looking for something sweet. Her favorite breakfast was pancakes because it gave her a reason to have maple syrup. If she was

eating on the run, it might be a cinnamon bun or a doughnut and coffee (sweetened). She kept drinking coffee most
of the day, and there was always some chocolate of some
kind around the office. She hardly had time to shop, prepare, and cook dinner—so she generally ate out.

Lindsey was a happy person, and it was fun talking with
her and hearing about her experiences. We looked over
some photos she had of herself going back 20 years; it was
interesting to see how she had changed, especially recently.
Once quite slender, she had developed a more barrel-shaped
appearance, with weight gain primarily around her chest
and belly. She joked about wanting to rearrange some of the
weight from her belly down to her hips and buttocks, where
she felt she needed more.

When I took a look at Lindsey's blood-test results, another pattern started to emerge. Her blood revealed that
she was borderline diabetic and had bad cholesterol levels.
A number of abnormalities surfaced, including elevated levels of C-reactive protein—a blood marker of inflammation.
Lindsey's level of triglycerides was also too high.

All of this added up to a dangerous situation, because
these are the markers of heart attack and stroke.

Lindsey knew she had to make changes. The good
news is that the timing was perfect. She was ready and just
needed to know what to do. That's when I explained more
about the Hunter/Farmer types.

Lindsey was a classic Hunter: she had developed an
addictive relationship to sugar, she had gained all of her
weight around the middle of her body in the chest and
abdomen, and she was prediabetic with a high risk of cardiovascular problems. All of her health issues had sprung
from overeating sugar and carbs.

Lindsey understood. Sugar was like a drug for her, a substance like alcohol that could also be addictive and damaging. She quickly committed to learning ways to eat a better diet.

The good news is that Lindsey left the Ranch like she was shot out of a cannon; she had a new lease on life, and a new way of thinking about eating and nutrition. And, she had remarkable success—during the next year, she lost 60 pounds! When she returned to Canyon Ranch for her one-year anniversary, she looked amazing. She was fit, slim, and energetic. Lindsey was especially thrilled when we repeated her blood work and found that everything had returned completely to normal.

❦ ❦ ❦

Lindsey's success is possible for all of us—including you—once we learn which type we are and which diet to follow.

Remember that Hunters and Farmers can be discerned in several ways: where they store fat, their ancestry and birth history, and the results of some simple blood tests. Let's take a closer look at what makes these two types unique, and find out which one best describes you.

❧ ❧ ❧

CHAPTER THREE

THE HUNTER/FARMER STORY

We've talked about the history of food, and the two types of people: Hunters and Farmers. But why are there two types of metabolisms that need two different diets? What accounts for these two types?

First, the idea of being a Hunter or a Farmer shouldn't be taken literally; I'm not talking about whether you actually hunt things or grow things in a garden. The terms apply to a new paradigm—a new way of thinking about eating and controlling weight. The terms are useful because they also explain in part the eating strategy that's best for you.

Hunters and Farmers are very different, and in some ways, opposite in their eating behaviors and food choices. As mentioned, Hunters are dependent on hunting animals or finding edible plants, fruits, and nuts. Farmers grow crops that can be stored to create a surplus that provides a dependable and readily available source of calories. The

Hunter's diet is more sporadic and depends on where and when food resources become available. Hunters are naturally more resistant to the effects of food shortages, as they're better able to maintain a steady blood-sugar level, or to use belly fat for immediate energy. Farmers are more sensitive to food shortages, as they become hypoglycemic—that is, they get low blood sugar—when they've gone just a few hours without food.

The most significant difference between Hunters and Farmers is that they have varying sensitivity to the hormone insulin. Hunters are *insulin resistant,* and Farmers are *insulin sensitive.*

Insulin Resistance and Insulin Sensitivity

Insulin is an important hormone made by the pancreas. Most people are aware of its primary effect, which is to lower blood sugar after a meal. That's true, because insulin is an energy storage hormone that allows our cells to take up nutrients flowing into the bloodstream after we eat. Insulin acts like a key that unlocks transport mechanisms on the surface of our cells, especially cells in our liver and muscles. Once unlocked, nutrients start to flow from the bloodstream into our cells, where they can be used for energy or for growth and repair.

Normally, after we eat, food is digested and broken down into its basic nutrient building blocks so that we can absorb and transport them. Carbohydrates are broken down into sugar (glucose), fats are broken down into fatty acids, and protein is broken down into amino acids. After a meal, levels of glucose, fatty acids (as triglycerides), and amino acids rise in the bloodstream. Insulin released from the pancreas acts as a receptor on the cells' surface that causes our cells to soak up the glucose. That's how insulin lowers blood sugar: it causes our cells to soak up the glucose from the bloodstream.

Lowering blood sugar is actually providing energy to our cells, because as the cells soak up glucose and other nutrients, they can turn that into energy.

The difference between Hunters and Farmers is how well their cells respond to signals from insulin. Farmers' cells are exquisitely sensitive to the effects of insulin; just a small amount of it released from the pancreas is enough to lower a Farmer's blood-sugar levels substantially. That's why Farmers are especially prone to low blood sugar—they are so sensitive to the effects of insulin that any excess amount is enough to drop blood sugar.

The reverse is true for Hunters, who are resistant to the effects of insulin. It takes more insulin to produce the same glucose-lowering effect. Hunters' liver cells and muscles don't respond as readily to insulin (they don't soak up as much glucose from the blood), so their blood-sugar levels stay relatively higher. That's why Hunters show two common findings on their blood tests: high glucose and high insulin. Worsening insulin resistance can develop into diabetes, especially if a Hunter gains weight, or sometimes just as a result of the aging process.

The sensitivity to insulin is the most important hallmark of Hunters and Farmers, and it can be measured with a fairly common office test called the glucose tolerance test (GTT). It's often done to check for diabetes and to see how someone handles carbohydrates.

Here's how the test is conducted: A baseline blood sample is drawn for glucose and insulin levels. Then you drink a sweet beverage containing 50 grams of glucose or dextrose, and blood tests are repeated after 30 minutes and 120 minutes.

A normal fasting blood-sugar level is between 75 and 100. Borderline fasting blood sugar is between 100 and 126. Blood sugar above 127 (fasting) is considered diabetic. Nonfasting blood sugars can go as high as 200 even under normal conditions, depending on what you ate.

Another way to monitor long-term blood-sugar levels is with the Hemoglobin A1c (A1c) Test, which measures the percentage of hemoglobin that has sugar attached. Optimal levels are below 6 percent, high levels are 7 percent and above. Here's a table with optimal values:

	Optimal	Borderline Risk	High Risk
Glucose	75–99	100–126	> 127
A1c	< 6.0%	6–7%	> 7.0%

The results of the glucose tolerance test explain how someone processes a glucose load, and separates the Hunters from the Farmers. For example, see the following graph:

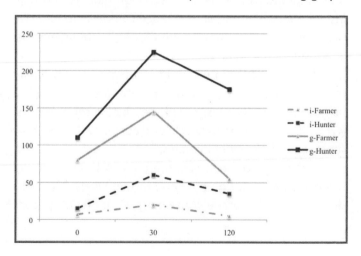

This graph shows that the Hunter type (in black) has both higher blood sugar (glucose; solid black line) and higher insulin levels (dotted black line) than the Farmer. The Hunter's glucose level often stayed above the normal range even two hours after the glucose drink (glucose should stay below 180, even after a meal). The Farmer's glucose level (solid gray line) was often below the normal range at two hours, with symptoms of hypoglycemia (low blood sugar) including shakiness, queasiness, and sweating.

Low blood sugar is considered less than 75. The test is very helpful to understand how the body can handle a fixed load of sugar. The only limitation is that during the test (two hours), you can't exercise because exercise lowers both glucose and insulin.

So the varying levels of glucose and insulin are characteristic of the Hunter and Farmer types, and the differences are explained by an individual's degree of insulin resistance or insulin sensitivity. Why would nature produce two distinct types, and why would they differ in their responsiveness to insulin? The answer may in part be due to *stress*.

The Stress Factor

Insulin resistance is, most likely, an adaptation to stress. Insulin-resistant Hunters may have been "programmed" in this way to help them survive in a stressful environment. For instance, in the historical Hunter's world, food is typically scarce, there is more time between meals, and life is more chaotic than the Farmer's. Assuming that crops are growing, Farmers have a bit more security. Their lifestyle provides the security of a stockpile of food, which allows them to devote time to activities other than finding food. They don't tend to be subjected to as much stress as Hunters; in fact, stress might be one of the contributing factors that can cause the Hunter-type metabolism.

Cortisol is the main stress hormone that is made in the adrenal glands. High cortisol levels are produced during the stress response, which also triggers an increase in the hunger for calorie-rich foods. This might explain why stress makes us crave sweets, and why Hunters might have a natural weakness for sweets, because they have higher cortisol levels.

Higher cortisol in Hunters may be part of the reason for some of the typical findings, including high blood sugar, high blood pressure, and abdominal weight gain. Those same physical changes can occur if non-Hunters are given supplemental cortisol or cortisone; they will slowly develop Hunter characteristics: higher glucose and insulin levels, as well as insulin resistance that can lead to belly fat, high blood pressure, and diabetes.

Everyone's cortisol level changes from minute to minute, hour to hour, and even day to day. But it usually follows a repeating pattern. Cortisol is generally highest first thing in the morning. It's one of the hormones involved in waking us up from sleep and getting us going for the day. By mid-morning the levels are falling and stay in the mid-range during the day. After dinner and before bed, levels reach their lowest as we prepare to sleep. Cortisol then remains low throughout the night until we arise in the morning and the cycle repeats.

Here's a graph of typical cortisol levels throughout the day (Hunters are the dashed line; Farmers the solid line):

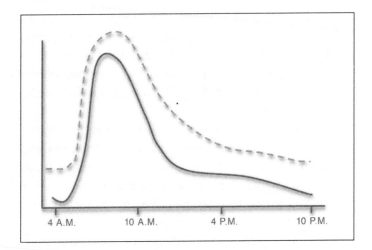

The Hunter pattern is typical of a stress response. It's also a similar profile seen with depression or anxiety. In other words, the Hunter shows similar results to someone under stress, with high cortisol levels and all its possible complications.

But it's oversimplistic to think that ordinary stress alone causes diabetes or even the Hunter's metabolism. The kind of stress that does is a longer-term, lifelong kind. In fact, there's a lot of evidence that the stress began before we were born—back when we were in our mother's womb. The evidence is found in what we've learned about birth weight.

Birth Weight

Birth weight is an important indicator of many things, including the stress of a newborn.

Any number of factors can cause stress during pregnancy —it's amazing that it all goes so well so often. But babies can be born tiny for many reasons, ranging from problems with the placenta to complications like prematurity. Most of these factors are not under our direct control. Others, like maternal smoking and poor nutrition, are. What's interesting is that our birth weight affects our risk for diabetes later in adulthood.

Normal birth weight is considered between 6.5 and 9.5 pounds. Smaller babies, and even babies in the lower end of the normal range, are more likely to develop the Hunter metabolism that can lead to diabetes later in life. The relationship seems to hold regardless of the reason for a baby's size at birth (except perhaps for small parents whose families typically have small babies; the smaller size is just normal for them).

It's not entirely clear how being a small baby can program your body toward being a Hunter. It's possible that the reverse is true; being a Hunter makes you a small baby. We don't know. But one theory is that the brain is actually in control. We know that the brain needs glucose. Unlike other organs, it can't burn fat or use protein for energy. Only glucose keeps the lights on. That's important when a baby is small, stressed, and trying to survive and grow. Small babies actually have to grow faster to catch up to where they should be for their age. Most often, they catch up by the time they turn one.

While the baby's body is growing so quickly, the brain needs to prevent the growing body from using up all available glucose, so the brain may program the rest of the body (and mainly the muscles) to become insulin resistant. If the muscles are insulin resistant, then they would leave more glucose behind to protect the brain's primary fuel source. It's just a theory, but the point is that birth weight is a factor in predicting the later development of diabetes and therefore of the Hunter type.

Of course we can't change what our birth weight was; it's just another factor to be aware of. But this might explain how stress adaptation begins for the Hunter even before birth. Naturally, Farmers can experience just as much stress as Hunters do; they just aren't programmed that way from birth.

Belly Fat and Hip Width

The effects of insulin resistance and high cortisol actually change the way our bodies look and behave. That's because insulin is a storage hormone, and cortisol makes us store that fat as belly fat. And belly fat is another pivotal difference between Hunters and Farmers.

High levels of insulin and cortisol lead to the typical apple shape of the Hunter. Lower levels of insulin and cortisol, typical of the Farmer, produce more subcutaneous fat—fat under the skin that can accumulate in a more evenly distributed way, which produces the typical Farmer shape, accentuating curves and skin folds.

The kind of belly fat that accumulates in Hunters is not just under the skin. It's actually located inside the abdominal cavity, surrounding and cushioning the internal organs such as the bowel, liver, kidneys, bladder, and so forth. Because of its location around these visceral organs, this type of belly fat is known as visceral fat.

Farmer fat is the fat you can "pinch"; the fat that's deep in the belly is the Hunter fat. Besides its location, Hunter fat has different effects than Farmer fat. Hunter fat is linked with higher levels of glucose and triglycerides in the blood because it is actually a gut organ that produces hormones that help regulate appetite and metabolism. Hunter fat releases hormones such as leptin, adiponectin, and ghrelin into the circulation around the gut organs and the liver, specifically.

The liver is pivotal in this story, producing and releasing glucose, triglycerides, and cholesterol particles according to signals it receives from the pancreas and other gut organs, including the visceral Hunter fat. Science is just starting to understand how the hormones produced by Hunter fat in the gut regulate our appetite and metabolism. What's clear is that Hunter fat is a bioactive organ releasing hormones that have effects on our blood sugar, cholesterol, and triglyceride levels.

One way to tell what kind of belly fat you have is to take a squeeze. Visceral fat is located below the muscle layer of the belly, while subcutaneous fat is located above the muscle layer. So if you tighten up your belly muscles as tight as you can and then squeeze the fat, what you're squeezing is subcutaneous Farmer fat. The rest is the visceral Hunter fat.

You probably have some of each; what's significant is which is predominant. One way to measure that is to compare the size of your belly to the size of your hips: the famous waist-hip ratio. The higher the number (waist divided by hips), the more your fat is belly fat—the more of a Hunter you are. A low waist-hip ratio represents the Farmer type.

But it's not just about the belly. Hip width can also help distinguish Hunters from Farmers. Farmers tend to have bigger, wider hips, compared with Hunters' relatively narrow hips. Hunter women typically have narrower hips giving them more of a boyish shape than Farmer women, who tend to have wider hips and buttocks.

The Farmer shape has become much more fashionable in recent years. In the past, slender, boyish-shaped anorectic models dominated the media; recently "Farmer figures" like Kim Kardashian and Jennifer Lopez have made the Farmer shape popular.

For men, hip width is also important. As a male Farmer gains weight, he will put on weight very evenly. His thighs and buttocks grow as fast as his belly and arms. His shape becomes wider and cylindrical, growing evenly.

By contrast, as a male Hunter gains weight, the pounds accumulate mainly in the belly and chest, but the hips, thighs, and legs stay relatively lean and narrow. Men who keep the same belt size as they gain weight are likely to be Hunters—their hips aren't growing; only their belly is, and that usually hangs over the belt, which is on the same notch as it was 15 years ago!

Now, there's no specific cutoff that's "good" or "bad" or Hunter or Farmer. People are all different sizes, so it's really the relative hip width for that individual. It's the width of the hips relative to the waist. It's the butt compared to the belly. That is a sensitive indicator of your Hunter/Farmer type.

Hip width is an easy way to separate Hunters and Farmers, and it's also another suggestion that your metabolism was programmed into your body from a very early age, probably before birth. Your body shape is one way to help you to determine your own personal dietary needs, at least in terms of macronutrients.

❧ ❧ ❧

The shape and physical characteristics of both Hunters and Farmers become accentuated when you gain weight. A slim Hunter and a slim Farmer are hard to tell apart. Even their blood results start looking more similar when a Hunter and Farmer lose weight.

The problems arise when you eat the wrong diet—for example, when a Hunter eats a Farmer diet, or a Farmer eats a Hunter diet. In those cases, you're likely to gain weight. And when you do gain weight, it tends to be either Hunter fat or Farmer fat, depending on your type.

Gaining weight accentuates the shape of a Hunter or Farmer, and it also accentuates the results of your blood tests. The reverse is also true: As you lose weight, the features of the Hunter or Farmer become less obvious and harder to tell apart. That's the success of the Hunter/Farmer Diet: Once you are on the right diet, weight, body shape, and blood results all start to normalize.

By now you should have a pretty good idea as to which type you probably are. To confirm your suspicions, please take the following quiz that highlights the differences between Hunters and Farmers. Here's how it works: For each trait, circle the closest response for you from either the Hunter column or the Farmer column. If you don't know the answer to the question, or it doesn't apply, you can leave it blank. The more responses you're able to fill in, the more accurate your result will be.

When you're finished, count the number of boxes you've circled in each column. If you've circled more responses in the Hunter column, then you are a Hunter. If you've circled more responses in the Farmer column, you are a Farmer. Let's get started!

TRAIT	HUNTER	FARMER
When I gain weight, it seems to go mostly to my:	Belly and/or chest	Hips, thighs, buttocks
My hips and buttocks are best described as:	Narrow and flat	Wide and rounded
My thighs are best described as:	Relatively thin	Thick
In a pool, I tend to float most like a:	Jellyfish, with my legs hanging down in the water	Surfboard, with my legs out straight
I have a substantial amount of cellulite:	Not really	Yes
My appetite:	I don't get hungry that often	I am hungry often
My birth weight was:	Less than seven pounds	Seven pounds or more
How I feel about sweets:	I crave them	I could take them or leave them
If I have a drink of alcohol, the next thing I'll probably want is:	Another drink	Something to eat
My HDL ("good") cholesterol level is:	Low, should be higher	Good; just right
My blood sugar (glucose)*:	100 or over	Below 100
My triglycerides*:	Over 150, fasting	Below 150
My A1c level*:	6 percent or less	Over 6 percent
My C-reactive protein level*:	Over 2 mg/L	2 mg/L or less
I have experienced symptoms of hypoglycemia**:	Not often	Yes, often

TRAIT	HUNTER	FARMER
Health conditions I've had or are prevalent in my family:	Cardiovascular diseases: heart disease, stroke, and diabetes	Cancer
I am more likely to get pain in my:	Back	Hips
My blood pressure tends to run:	Borderline high or high	Low

*Without medications (if you are already on medications for cholesterol, triglycerides, blood sugar, or inflammation, your numbers may not apply). You may use blood-test results from before you started on medications, if those are available.

**Hypoglycemia, or low blood sugar, causes symptoms of irritability, weakness, queasiness, lightheadedness or dizziness, and perspiration.

Note: Most people will have a majority of factors in one column or the other. It's possible to have an even split, although not likely, as these traits track together. An even amount of both means a perfect blend of Hunter/Farmer traits, in which case you'll have to eat meals from both plans. But again, very few people will have an even score, especially if you're able to respond to all of the questions.

※ ※ ※

So now you know whether you are a Hunter, made to eat a Hunter diet, or a Farmer in need of a Farmer diet. Let's begin with Hunters and discuss what they need to eat in order to lose weight and become healthier.

🍂 🍂 🍂

CHAPTER FOUR

THE HUNTER DIET

I'm used to seeing Hunter patients when they're in some kind of crisis: They just had a heart scare; their blood pressure has climbed rapidly; or they flunked a company physical due to their weight, blood sugar, or cholesterol. Perhaps they hit an all-time high number on the scale, or they had a parent suffer an illness that potentially could have been prevented.

These Hunters come to Canyon Ranch for a complete checkup and for help in losing weight and regaining their health. The good news is that by the time they've made it to my office, they are almost always ready for change, and that makes my job easier. It reminds me of the old joke: How many psychiatrists does it take to change a light bulb? Just one, but the light bulb has to want to change.

The first part in helping that light bulb change is by explaining the Hunter type and the Hunter diet. Once people understand more about what to eat and why, it becomes much easier to make the right choices in any situation.

If you are a Hunter, as mentioned previously, you have some natural traits that were designed to help you survive under conditions of foraging and finding food. Perhaps the most important is the Hunter's ability to go for longer periods of time without eating. A Hunter is naturally better adapted to conditions where food is scarce, and where larger "feasts" are separated by longer periods of leaner times. The Hunter is adapted to store energy in the belly, where it can more easily be drawn upon during the lean times when food is scarce.

Hunters can switch back and forth very quickly between using blood sugar for energy, then using abdominal fat for energy if blood-sugar supplies get low. Hunters also maintain a higher average blood-sugar level than Farmers. That higher blood sugar can provide energy longer, and sustain the Hunter during times when food is less available.

The problems arise when a Hunter starts eating like a Farmer, which pushes the Hunter farther along the road toward diabetes and obesity. Hunters have problems metabolizing sugar. It's not so much of a problem if you're an actual hunter, because you're eating meat and fish and a few leaves and berries—foods without much sugar. What a Hunter can't handle well is the sugar—or any load of food that is converted to sugar such as grains, breads, pasta, corn, and starchy vegetables like potatoes, turnips, parsnips, and squash.

The primary objective in diabetes is controlling high blood sugar (glucose). A fasting blood sugar above 126 milligrams per deciliter is the cutoff for the diagnosis of diabetes. (*Please note:* For the purposes of this book, the use of the term *diabetes* always refers to type 2 diabetes, not type 1.) Normally your fasting blood sugar should be less than 100 milligrams per deciliter. What's typical of (type 2) diabetics is that they run a higher than average blood-sugar level throughout the day. Long-term measures of blood sugar (called hemoglobin A1c, or just A1c) are also elevated above 6 percent, confirming higher average blood-sugar levels.

A diabetic's blood-sugar level shoots up even higher after a meal and it stays up longer. The problem is when the blood sugar shoots up even higher than that. When diabetes worsens and blood sugar continues to climb, then damage to the organs (the eyes, kidneys, nerves, and heart) occurs and accumulates. The main goal of treatment is to control the blood-sugar level, because that minimizes the complications of diabetes.

This reminds me of one of my favorite patients, Brian. When I first met him, he was 42 years old and had come in for a checkup at the Ranch. Brian was barely middle-aged, yet he had been diabetic for six years. He was from a well-to-do family, but he had been born with disabilities and had grown up in a group-home setting. Despite his challenges, he was one of the most positive, energetic, and happy people I know. Brian had always received excellent health care, but he inevitably ended up on a longer and longer list of medications to treat a variety of ailments, mostly springing from his diabetes. He was taking insulin, in addition to several pills to control his blood sugar. He was also taking medication for his blood pressure, cholesterol, triglycerides, and thyroid, as well as something for acid reflux and something else for sleep.

It's a common story: As we age and see more doctors, we usually end up on more and more medications. Some are prescribed just to offset the side effects from the others.

I can understand how it happens, but it always disturbs me to see such long lists of prescription drugs; and I'm always trying to think about which ones could be eliminated, in which order, and what alternatives there might be.

One of the first things on the hit list for Brian was insulin. Not only did I want to get him off of it, but he also wanted that very much. I explained that it was fully possible as long as he agreed to change some things about his diet and make an effort to lose weight. In his always-positive style, Brian flashed a huge grin and declared that he was going to do it!

The good news was that Brian was in the perfect place to learn how to make those changes successfully. He understood the Hunter diet right away, and he asked the right questions: "That means no more bagels and doughnuts, right?"

Brian really wanted to stop his insulin because he didn't like having to take the shots, but he was also starting to experience major complications: his kidneys were showing signs of damage, as was his vision, and his sense of touch in his hands and feet was deteriorating. He was getting burning, "sandpapery" feelings in his feet and toes that are typical of nerve damage. All of these issues could be attributed to his diabetes—specifically, by his blood sugar being too high.

Brian spent a week at Canyon Ranch and much of that was teaching him about the Hunter diet. We immediately started him on his new diet, and he was checking his blood-sugar readings twice a day. He also took in some exercise classes and a massage after dinner. This was a great way to get healthy as far as Brian was concerned. We then agreed that he would come back in three months to see how it was going.

Brian was filled with a new sense of control over his health and well-being. Three months later when he was back in my office, he was flashing his huge grin and showing off his slimmer body! The results were fantastic. Over the three months, Brian lost around 20 pounds and his blood-sugar readings were dramatically improved—so good that we were able to stop his insulin injections altogether. Not only that, but we were also able to reduce the medications he was taking for his blood pressure, cholesterol, and triglycerides. The best part was that Brian felt a lot better—he had much more energy, as well as less discomfort in his feet.

How had he done all this?

The key was sharply reducing grains and grain products from his diet, while finding substitutes that Brian enjoyed, such as beans, berries, nuts, seeds, and fruits, along with good protein sources from fish, poultry, and lean meats. We found a food service that cooked healthy meals according to the right specifications that Brian could keep in the fridge and reheat. He would bring one to work and have it for lunch instead of going for a couple slices of pizza or some other fast food. Brian liked the healthy food, and he really liked how he felt, especially not having to take as much medication.

Brian also learned a vital trick that helped him control his blood-sugar levels. By checking his blood sugar with the finger-prick glucose monitor, we saw that his readings often spiked in the morning after breakfast, and again in the afternoon following lunch. Brian started taking a 15-minute walk—once in the morning and once in the afternoon—and he noticed that just this simple activity would bring his blood-sugar level down.

In addition, he learned an important point about exercise: it uses up blood sugar and brings down blood-sugar levels. One of the best ways for Hunters to control their blood sugar is with moderate exercise. Most people think that it helps you lose weight because it burns calories. But more important is that exercise helps bring down both blood-sugar and insulin levels, and that's what is really helpful for Hunters.

In other words, Hunters' naturally higher blood-sugar and insulin levels can be controlled with exercise more effectively than with medications.

Historically, the Hunter's diet was naturally low in sugar, starches, and grains. You can't hunt grains, and there weren't a lot of foods that would raise their blood sugar that much. So their standard diet didn't exacerbate an already high blood sugar. Having a slightly higher blood sugar may have also given Hunters the extra-quick energy they might need for hunting prey or foraging food. The ability of the Hunter to store a readily accessible source of energy (belly fat) that also acted to help suppress appetite was a helpful survival trait. But, as we now know, the problems begin when a diabetic gets too much belly fat. The same trait that can help a prediabetic Hunter survive in the savanna becomes a huge health risk when there's too much of it.

Belly fat is also a big risk factor for heart disease, and being shaped more like an apple is a well-known association with heart attack and stroke. One reason is the effect that too much belly fat has on our cholesterol and triglyceride levels. Excess belly fat leads to low HDL cholesterol, and low levels are a risk for cardiovascular disease.

✿ ✿ ✿

Hunters usually have no problem skipping a meal. Their natural ability to maintain blood-sugar levels means that meals can be farther apart. No doubt you've heard all the popular advice to the contrary: that breakfast is the most important meal of the day, and everyone should eat a big breakfast. That's not necessarily true for Hunters, however, who are less likely to feel hungry first thing in the morning.

A recent study from Germany busted the myth about breakfast being the most vital meal. Researchers found that the calories eaten at breakfast did not reduce calories eaten subsequently during the day. In fact, the more calories that were eaten at breakfast, the more calories the person ate the entire day.

So if you're a Hunter and you're not hungry at breakfast time, you shouldn't feel compelled to eat something. Skipping breakfast isn't a bad strategy, especially since so many breakfast foods aren't ideal for Hunters. (A good breakfast might be eggs, but we'll get into the Hunter's specific diet plan soon.)

The goal of the Hunter is to keep blood-sugar levels from spiking. Breakfast foods like cereal, breads, dough-nuts, croissants, and pancakes are quickly absorbed from the intestine as sugar after brief digestion in the stomach. Those foods will cause a Hunter's blood sugar to spike ex-tremely high, because they're simple carbs that are quickly converted to sugar. A stack of pancakes and maple syrup contains a lot of sugar, and a Hunter's blood sugar can rise into the range of diabetes after that kind of breakfast.

If you're a Hunter, right now you're probably thinking that you wish you were a Farmer because pancakes and maple syrup, a doughnut or bagel, and a bowl of oat-meal with brown sugar are among your all-time favorites. But that's how most Hunters become overweight. It's the pathologic relationship with sugar that has caused all of the problems—the weight gain, the belly fat, the inflammation, the fatigue, and the abnormal blood results. For many Hunters, it's beyond a relationship . . . it's an addiction.

And Hunters are especially prone to sugar addiction. The reason has to do with how sugar affects brain hormones like serotonin. Serotonin is the "feel good" hormone, elevating mood and sense of calm. Antidepressants such as Prozac and similar drugs work by boosting serotonin levels, which boosts mood and calms nerves.

Sugar has a similar, although perhaps lesser, effect also boosting serotonin levels. Hunters may be particularly susceptible to sugar because studies show that Hunters have lower levels of serotonin compared to Farmers. Hunters may be craving more than just the calories that come from sugar; they're also craving the serotonin surge that makes you feel so good.

Doctors began prescribing serotonin-boosting antidepressants in the 1990s, mostly after the weight-loss combo medication "phen-fen" (phentermine-fenfluramine) was pulled from the market because of links with heart-valve problems. But the use of Prozac for aiding weight loss has continued to some degree. Of course nothing works for everybody, and it's possible that your Hunter/Farmer type could predict whether you might respond to Prozac or other serotonin-blocking medication.

However, it's not all entirely about serotonin. Myriad brain chemicals are used to transmit different emotions and physiologic states. There is a complicated interplay of a variety of brain chemicals and hormones involved in emotions like love, pleasure, and joy. Some of the known chemical signals include adrenaline, noradrenaline, dopamine, serotonin, oxytocin, and acetylcholine. There are many more, and new brain chemicals are still being discovered. It's possible that drugs of the future may target other brain hormones or receptors to reduce appetite or regulate weight.

Strategies to boost serotonin and other so-called feel-good brain hormones are especially suited for Hunters. Some of the other proven ways of boosting serotonin include exercise, getting proper sleep, laughter, and smiling . . . just to name a few.

Cutting Carbs

The single most important lesson for a Hunter who wants to lose weight is to learn to control excessive sugar and carbohydrate consumption. That's not easy, especially if you've developed a sugar addiction. Chances are you may already have experience getting rid of an addiction—smoking, alcohol, coffee, chocolate, diet pills, energy drinks and sodas, gambling, or even shopping. There are a lot of possible things to which one can become addicted! A lot of them you can give up altogether, but you can't really give up carbs completely. Even foods like beans or fruit have some carbs, athough they aren't such a problem as quicker carbs—those that show up as a spike of glucose in your bloodstream.

Remember, carbs should be considered in a supporting role, not as the lead act in your diet. The optimal amount of carbs varies from person to person. Someone with full-blown diabetes should be ingesting fewer carbs than someone with a normal blood-sugar reading. The severity of the problem usually dictates the need for restriction. The higher your blood sugar, the more you need to restrict carbs.

Blood tests might be helpful. Very high glucose (>150) or triglyceride levels (>400) indicate a need to severely restrict, if not eliminate, any sweets or refined carbohydrates. Moderately high glucose (>125) or triglyceride (>200) levels require moderate to marked carbohydrate restriction, and mildly high glucose (>100) or triglyceride (>150) levels require milder carbohydrate restriction. Optimal levels of blood glucose are between 65 and 95, and "normal" levels are below 100. Optimal triglyceride levels (fasting, unmedicated) are less than 100 mg/dl and "normal" levels are below 150 mg/dl.

A Hunter has found the right diet when fasting glucose drops below 100 and triglycerides are below 150. Those can be used as a guide of progress and success. Your doctor can prescribe a glucose meter so you can test your own fasting blood sugar if you're so inclined. (Triglycerides require a blood test at a clinic or your doctor's office.)

When it comes to cutting carbs, here are a few tips. First, it helps to exercise, which raises serotonin much like carbs do. Going through carb withdrawal means feeling uncomfortable with lower serotonin levels; and you may also feel sluggish, depressed, achy, or irritable. Physical activity helps by boosting brain serotonin levels; you'll notice an immediate improvement in your energy level, mood, and outlook right away. People going through carb withdrawal should exercise regularly.

Not all carbs need to be restricted or eliminated. As mentioned, there are many sources of carbohydrates, including healthy ones such as beans, nuts, and seeds, as well as fruits and vegetables. Those sources either contain little carbohydrates, or release them so slowly that they're low glycemic—that is, they won't spike your blood sugar. Keep in mind that sweets, starches, and grains are different.

Hunters' metabolism to deal with. The quicker any food is converted to sugar, the worse it is for Hunters in any quantity. Thus, milled grains like cereals, white flour, white rice, and refined grains of all kinds are the biggest offenders, since they're converted more quickly to pure sugar, namely *glucose.* The bottom line is that large portions of refined and "white" grains should be minimized, if not eliminated, in the Hunter's diet.

Likewise, sweets and sugary foods are especially damaging, requiring very little digestion for immediate conversion to glucose. Large portions can spike a Hunter's blood sugar for several hours. Prolonged high blood sugar begins to cause microscopic damage to the blood vessels, the eyes, nerve endings, and so forth, accelerating the progress to diabetes.

Hunters need some intake of glucose, of course. Without a regular supply, our bodies will use protein sources and convert those to glucose. Hunters' glucose sources should provide a slow, steady release into the bloodstream, so low-glycemic foods are ideal. Beans and berries, for example, are a low-glycemic source of glucose that won't spike blood-sugar levels. Likewise, most vegetables also provide low-glycemic sources of glucose; the sugar content of vegetables is low and released slowly without spiking blood sugar. Beans and berries are high in fiber, which helps to slow their release of glucose while providing us the added benefits of more fiber.

Most fruits are sweeter and capable of delivering too much sugar, especially when it's concentrated as in fruit or dried fruits. The good news is that fruit sugar (fructose) requires conversion to glucose to produce blood so eating fruit is actually low glycemic. However, only true in small quantities, as with eating fruit,

Those sources of carbs are quickly turned into glucose and spike blood glucose and insulin levels. This is especially true of the refined or "white" grains including white flour, white rice, white pasta, and so on.

If you've been a habitual user of sugar, sweets, and carbs for their mood-boosting effects and you plan to break the habit, you ought to prepare as best you can. You'll need to boost your own serotonin levels as much as possible. In addition to exercise, it's also important to maintain a healthy vitamin D level. Be sure to get some sun exposure (no sunburns, please!) or take a vitamin D supplement. Most people could benefit from taking 2,000 IU of vitamin D3 daily, unless you get regular sun exposure.

The amino acid tryptophan is a precursor for serotonin synthesis, so it's important to have enough tryptophan on board. Meats are good sources; you've probably heard of the "turkey-dinner effect," because turkey is a good source of tryptophan. It's also available in supplements in the form of 5-HTP, which is sometimes recommended for help with mood or sleep.

Physical touch can help, too. Intimacy and sexuality boost serotonin and other feel-good hormones. Massage is an excellent way to lessen some of the pain of going through carb withdrawal. Acupuncture can also play a tremendous role in stimulating the relaxation response and positive energy flow.

Dark chocolate seems to benefit some people, but for many, it's very difficult to eat just a little. In fact, sometimes it's better not to start at all, unless you can truly limit portion size. Chocolate can become another addiction.

Withdrawal is a sort of agitated discomfort, so anything that calms the nerves is helpful. Try herbal teas, hot tubs, candles and aromas, massages and body treatments, all of which can help soften the edge of carbohydrate with-drawal.

Some people prefer to go cold turkey and suffer all of the withdrawal, agitation, and cravings at once, rather than stretching out the misery for days or weeks. In my practice I have noticed that it takes two to three weeks for most people to cut their carbohydrate addiction if they follow the cold-turkey route. The good news is that once you've successfully cut out quick carbs, the craving for them goes down, so it's easier to stay away from them once they're out of your system.

※ ※ ※

Not every Hunter needs to eliminate carbs—some just need to reduce. This depends on how severe the effects are and how your blood tests look. Hunters should always consider the *quantity* of carbs. Portion size is key. I'd worry less about a teaspoon of sugar in a cup of coffee, which is only about 20 calories, compared with a plate of pasta or a piece of pie, which can be hundreds.

One simple way to know the quantity of carbs is by counting up the calories in whatever you're eating. Carbs provide 4 calories per gram, or about 113 calories per ounce. For alcohol, figure on 7 carb calories per gram of alcohol for pure alcohol, or about half that for 100 proof vodka, for example. A 1.5-ounce shot of 70-proof vodka would contain about 85 calories. Wine provides around 20 calories per ounce. A typical 5-ounce glass of red or white wine is about 100 calories of carbs.

A slice of bread, depending on the size and its ingredients, would usually have between 20 and 40 grams of carbs, or about 80 to 160 calories of carbs per slice. A plate of pasta at a restaurant can contain as much as 600 to 800 calories of carbs.

Becoming carb savvy is an important skill for the Hunter. It's wise to know how many carbs are in common foods and dishes, as that will help you make the best choices in any situation.

By the way, the biggest benefit to Hunters in cutting back on carbs is the immediate improvement in energy. It's often not until you get off the carbs that you realize how much they were negatively affecting your energy and disposition.

What Should Hunters Eat?

So what is the best diet for a Hunter? Since y
that the main trait of the Hunter is high blo
then the ideal diet should be low in sugar and
blood sugar (like grains). The Hunter diet is
low-carbohydrate diet.

That doesn't mean this is a carnivore o
It just means that while Hunters have carb
erance, they are relatively better at hand
tein. The ideal diet would be similar to v
consumed: an actual hunting-and-gath
cluded game but also fruits, nuts, roo
and leaves.

What wasn't part of our prin
gatherer diet were grains and the
tered the human diet roughly 1
and their derivatives are among
foods. Concentrated forms of
corn syrup and alcohol, whic

itself. In more concentrated forms, such as high-fructose corn syrup, sweetened fruit juices, and large portions of dried fruits, the amount of fructose is high enough to raise blood-glucose levels significantly.

Another great source of calories for Hunters is nuts. Very low glycemic in their release of carbohydrates, they provide high amounts of predominantly monounsaturated fats, which are considered healthful. Nuts are also a good source of fiber and antioxidants (selenium and vitamin E, for example), as well as some minerals like calcium and zinc. In addition, seeds provide healthy fats, proteins, fiber, and antioxidants.

Fish is an important part of the Hunter's diet, providing an excellent source of protein and healthy omega-3 fats without spiking blood sugar. The best fish for regular consumption are smaller-sized ones such as salmon, mackerel, char, herring, sardines, sole, trout, tilapia, and shellfish. Bigger fish like swordfish, tuna (except "chunk light"), tilefish, and sea bass should be saved for rare occasions. Those larger fish are higher (perhaps too high) in environmental toxins like PCBs, dioxins, pesticides, residues, and heavy metals, compared with smaller fish that are lower on the food chain. Fish should be on the menu at least twice a week for their health benefits and cardiovascular disease prevention.

Being on the Hunter diet means that it's generally okay to eat foods that you could kill or forage. Most people immediately think of a steak, but remember that hunters didn't exactly hunt cows. Cows appeared much later, after domestication took hold. The game that our ancestors were after was different from today's livestock. Back then it was antelope, buffalo, or even mammoths—definitely gamier and leaner than today's beef.

Even today there's a clear difference between eating elk or venison, say, than a T-bone or NY strip. That being said, there's probably also some value in grass-fed/free-range beef compared with grain-fed. It matters what our food has been eating, because it eventually becomes part of us. Free-range and grass-fed animals or game animals have fewer toxins and a healthier composition of fat than mass-produced meat from corn-fed cows.

The point is that meat is fine for Hunters, but leaner, free-range meats are probably better for regular consumption. The same could be said of poultry and fowl in general, whether it's chicken, turkey, duck, pheasant, quail, squab, grouse, and so forth.

One of the best Hunter foods is eggs. The original low-glycemic food, they are high in complete protein and very low in saturated fat. Eggs are the perfect food. However, many people are afraid to eat them because of their cholesterol: they have about 250 milligrams in each yolk, which is why many often eat just the egg whites. But the yolks contain omega-3 fats (even more in "omega eggs" and other free-range eggs), and they also contain many other vital nutrients—they are one of the best sources of choline, a compound that's an important nutrient for brain function.

Studies show that eating a couple of whole eggs every day is not likely to raise our cholesterol level. The average person with a blood cholesterol level of 200 mg/dl already has 40 eggs' worth of cholesterol in his or her bloodstream. And cholesterol is in every cell of the body, not just in the bloodstream. Our bodies manufacture around 3,000 milligrams of cholesterol daily for its use in cell membranes and hormone production. Eggs are especially low in saturated fat, so their net effect is neutral in terms of raising blood cholesterol. So eating a couple of eggs will not raise your cholesterol, and they are an excellent choice for the Hunter, as at only 75 calories apiece, they're a total bargain when it comes to low-glycemic nutrition.

Dairy products in general are also suitable in the Hunter diet. They do contain some sugar (lactose), but except for sweetened dairy products (such as ice cream, custards, and puddings), they are fairly low glycemic. Dairy is a good source of complete protein, too. Low-fat and nonfat options are widely available, but beware of added sweeteners. Nonfat yogurt might be fine, but not necessarily the syrup and jam at the bottom, for instance.

The Hunter has a wide range of options. Low-glycemic foods with elimination or limitation of refined grains and processed sweets is the cardinal rule. The degree to which you are able to limit these is proportional to your success with dieting.

The speed with which you eat is also a factor; it might take a half hour to sip a cup of tea or coffee, but only five minutes (or less) to eat an entire slice of pie. That surge of sugar has a much bigger and worse effect on your blood-sugar and insulin levels. Slower intake of carbs is better than faster intake. Here is a partial summary of the best foods to include, reduce, and avoid in the Hunter's diet:

Best Foods for Hunters	Foods to Limit	Foods to Avoid
Fish	Cereals	White bread
Poultry	Whole-grain bread	White pasta
Lean meats	Whole-grain pasta	White rice
Eggs	Potatoes	Cake
Non-starchy vegetables	Corn	Cookies
Berries	Bananas	Candy
Nuts	Juice	Sweetened cereals
Fruits	Ice cream	Sugary soft drinks
Beans and legumes	Dark chocolate	Sports drinks
Soy	Dried fruit	Rice milk
Dairy foods	Watermelon	Sugar, honey

❧ ❧ ❧

CHAPTER FIVE

THE FARMER DIET

As opposed to Hunters with high blood sugar, Farmers typically have low blood sugar—they are more likely to become hypoglycemic. Farmers also get hungry more often during the day, and if they ignore those hunger pangs, their blood sugar starts to dive and they can become hypoglycemic fairly quickly.

Low blood sugar, oddly, doesn't always make you feel hungry; more likely, you might feel queasy or even nauseous. Your legs might feel weak, your hands a little shaky, your thinking gets a bit fuzzy, and your decision making is a challenge. You might even get a little sweaty. It doesn't feel good; and if it lasts long, you're likely to be completely washed out and might need a nap to recover. These are familiar symptoms for those who have experienced this condition fairly often.

The solution for low blood sugar, of course, is to eat something to bring your level back up. One of the best picks is some form of carbohydrate—anything that provides sugar to raise the level in your blood. Eating a small amount of carbs is enough to quickly counteract hypogly-cemia, as long as you don't wait too long before eating; then the effects are longer lasting. People with a Farmer metabolism are not good at going for lengthy periods without eating.

The good news is that the Farmer metabolism is well suited to the Farmer diet, where grains are readily available to help maintain blood-sugar and energy levels. Recently, grains have been receiving bad press; most people consider foods like bread and pasta overly fattening. While it's true that Hunters need to limit or avoid them, it's certainly not true for those with the Farmer metabolism; they need carbs to keep their glucose and energy steady. And this is the foundation of the Farmer diet: a low-fat, grain-based meal plan that helps boost blood-sugar levels and prevent hypoglycemia.

The tendency for hypoglycemia is the hallmark of the Farmer metabolism, but there are also other common features of Farmers. One is the tendency to store fat under the skin—subcutaneous fat as opposed to Hunters, who have more abdominal, or visceral fat. As mentioned, as Farmers gain weight, it tends to be evenly distributed. The hips, thighs, and buttocks grow in size as do the arms and trunk, but the overall shape is generally maintained—unlike Hunters who primarily gain in the belly. Female Farmers retain their hourglass shape, and male Farmers get stockier and have a more cylindrical shape.

The accumulation of subcutaneous Farmer fat is similar to the way in which seals might keep a layer of blubber under their skin to keep warm in cold water. One interesting difference between Hunters and Farmers is how they float. Farmers float like a board: legs up high, toes out of the water. This is because the subcutaneous layer of fat is also in the legs, making them float up high in the water along with the rest of the body. On the other hand, Hunters float like jellyfish: belly up high, legs dangling down like tentacles.

Another result of the deposition of subcutaneous fat for Farmers is the layer of thick fat on the thighs and buttocks. This can sometimes become rippled and lumpy, leading to the very common appearance of cellulite in overweight Farmers. (Hunters are generally spared from cellulite.) Storing fat (subcutaneous energy) in the buttocks and thighs is typical of the Farmer, and this defines their body shape.

Let's take a closer look at Farmers' blood. We already know that they have low blood sugar compared to Hunters, and that they are far more sensitive to insulin. Because of this sensitivity, just a small amount of insulin released by the pancreas can lead to hypoglycemia. And even the sight or the thought of food can be enough to trigger a hypoglycemic reaction in Farmers. If you're a Farmer, you might have a lot of trouble resisting eating something after watching a tempting TV commercial about food.

Fortunately, Farmers have higher HDL ("good") cholesterol; they also have much lower triglycerides than Hunters. Both of these traits probably reflect how the Farmer's liver responds to the effects of insulin. Small amounts of insulin have powerful effects on the liver and largely determine the levels of HDL cholesterol and triglycerides in the blood. In addition, it's not uncommon for Farmers to have high total cholesterol *and* high LDL or "bad" cholesterol. In other words, Farmers often have high levels of both good and bad cholesterol at the same time. Again, that has to do with the way in which the Farmer's liver produces those cholesterol packets, and that's largely influenced by insulin.

Another common finding is that Farmers tend to have lower levels of inflammation, or CRP (C-reactive protein) levels. CRP and inflammation are now recognized as important factors that can worsen heart disease and contribute to diabetes and stroke, among other diseases. Because of their naturally lower level of inflammation, Farmers are less prone to heart disease, stroke, and diabetes.

The main reason why Farmers can easily gain weight is that they are subconsciously but deliberately protecting themselves against hypoglycemia.

❧ ❧ ❧

A perfect example is Blanche, a lovely 45-year-old patient of mine. Blanche was positive, energetic, and quite health conscious: She was a fitness buff and enjoyed dance classes, Pilates, and yoga. Always on the go, she was constantly multitasking, taking care of her family, cooking, shopping, working as a real-estate broker, and even volunteering for her church and a couple of charities.

For somebody doing so much and keeping so busy, you would think Blanche would be very thin, but she actually struggled with her weight. She knew all the things she was supposed to be doing with her diet and believed she should be thin, but somehow the more she tried to lose weight, the more weight she seemed to gain. Blanche explained that every diet made her feel tired and deprived, and even though she was trying to cut back, she'd find herself eating a half jar of peanuts in front of the TV at night, downing a double mocha soy latte in the afternoon, or devouring a pint of Ben & Jerry's ice cream before bed. The more she tried to diet and restrict herself, the more out of control she felt in giving in to impulsive eating.

It wouldn't take long before she realized that she was doing more harm than good in depriving herself with dieting, and she just went back to her usual way of eating. But in the process she had gained 25-plus pounds and would give almost anything to lose them.

Listening to Blanche tell her story of struggling with her weight reminded me of watching a movie on fast-forward. Blanche did everything fast. She talked fast, walked fast, moved fast, and ate fast. She was often the first one finished at the table, and she said she had always eaten fast. She attributed it to growing up in a family with four brothers; if she didn't eat fast, she might not get to eat at all! Of course it had been many years since she had to compete for food, but the habit was deeply ingrained.

Blanche also thought that part of the problem was how busy she was; she had so much to do that she had to eat quickly to save time. She rarely had a moment to relax over a meal, and even when she did, she still struggled to slow herself down. She could sip a glass of wine for an hour, but her food usually disappeared quickly.

The good news was that Blanche exercised regularly. After breakfast, she jog-walked three miles every morning around a track at her neighborhood high school and took a yoga or Pilates class two or three days a week. She and her family often took hiking or walking vacations, and went skiing in the winter. When Blanche came to Canyon Ranch, she'd take her morning walk and three or four exercise classes a day.

Blanche had learned that she needed to exercise daily, not just to keep her weight under control, but to also help clear her head. Physical activity was a great stress reliever, and she felt better when she worked out. Despite exercising regularly, however, it didn't seem to help her lose weight.

The scale just wasn't dropping—in fact, it was slowly creeping upward. This was incredibly frustrating because she was trying to do all the right things . . . but not having any success.

Spending time with Blanche led me to realize that she was a typical Farmer. The first clue was her shape: while small in stature at 5'3", Blanche had very noticeable and shapely curves—wide hips, a narrow waist, and thick thighs. She clearly tended to gain weight mostly in the hips, thighs, and buttocks.

Her blood work confirmed the Farmer pattern: low blood sugar (hers was 71 on a "normal" range between 75 and 99); high cholesterol—both HDL and LDL (with especially high HDL); low triglycerides (45); and low C-reactive protein (inflammation).

Blanche reported feeling hungry often during the day. Sometimes she'd feel famished by lunchtime, especially when she had done more exercise that morning. On days when she was busy and couldn't get to lunch until 1:30 or 2:00, she was beyond hungry and often felt exhausted, shaky, queasy, and weak. Blanche had learned to keep some string cheese and crackers in her desk drawer for emergencies when she wasn't able to get to lunch on time, or if she was working late.

She usually had cereal or oatmeal in the morning, along with some fruit and juice before her walk. Afterward, she mixed up a protein smoothie with bananas or berries and yogurt; she might have some nuts or a PowerBar on the way to work. I also learned that Blanche's thoughts during the day were often centered on food. She was always thinking about what she was going to bring to snack on, where she was going for lunch, and what she was planning for dinner. This behavior is typical of Farmers, as most are unconsciously (or consciously) obsessed with food because they have all experienced, at one time or another, low blood sugar.

Preventing and protecting against low blood sugar is a top priority item for Farmers, whether it's conscious or subconscious. The result is that they often learn two problematic eating behaviors: eating too fast and eating too much. If Farmers go too long without eating, blood-sugar levels start dropping. When they finally get food, they are desperate to bring their blood sugar back up and the natural reaction is to wolf down their meal.

The classic example is going out for dinner. By the time Farmers are seated and the waiter takes their order, they're hungry and their blood sugar is dropping. That's when many Farmers will do the wrong thing and eat two or three rolls or pieces of bread waiting for the meal to arrive; they just can't wait. Of course, once the entrée comes out, they're already full! They've restored their blood sugar by eating bread, and the dinner is now too many additional calories. And that quickly puts on weight.

When Farmers eat too fast, they also miss the usual cues of feeling full or satisfied. It takes a certain amount of time for the food, once swallowed, to actually be digested and appear in the bloodstream as energy (glucose). Eating too quickly leads to overeating. By the time blood sugar is restored and appetite is satisfied, most have already eaten more than enough, and the surplus is stored as fat.

For similar reasons, the Farmer has also learned to overeat. A full stomach is a good insurance policy against hypoglycemia. One surefire way to delay the next drop in blood sugar is to pack your stomach full of food. When you overeat, your stomach acts like a reservoir of calories that can last for a few hours. Farmers subconsciously overeat in order to protect themselves from hypoglycemia, which is why so many feel stuffed or like they've overeaten during a meal.

Those two problematic eating behaviors—eating too fast and eating too much—are the biggest hurdles for Farmers to overcome in their struggle to lose weight. The solution is to correct their problem eating behavior with two new strategies: eating more often and eating more slowly.

When I explained this to Blanche, I could see that she was getting it. It all made sense to her. She said it explained so much about her relationship with food, going back all the way to when she was a young woman.

Farmers like Blanche need to eat much more often, and in smaller quantities, just enough to restore blood sugar and keep energy levels up. Blanche learned that all she might need was a handful of granola, some carrot juice, or a few nuts every hour or two.

Blanche took my advice, and by eating more often, she never felt the deprivation she usually experienced while dieting. She still ate three meals, but they were smaller because her appetite was under control. Over the course of the day, although she was eating more often, she was eating less, because she had escaped the cycle of eating too fast and too much. She felt more in control of her eating than ever before.

For the first time Blanche also lost weight successfully! She was both thrilled and surprised to lose 15 pounds and three inches from her hips in just a few weeks without feeling the usual deprivation or suffering of dieting.

❧ ❧ ❧

The goal of the Farmer is to eat less over the day while keeping blood sugar levels from dropping. The best foods for boosting blood sugar are grains, since they're converted into blood sugar with digestion. And the best grains for Farmers are whole grains, such as whole wheat and whole oats. Whole grains, as opposed to refined grains like white flour, provide a steadier stream of glucose into the Farmer's system because they have more fiber, which helps control the release of sugar. The next best way to help support the Farmer's blood-sugar levels is to eat protein, since it can also be turned into glucose.

The last choice to help maintain blood sugar is food high in fat such as fried items, salad dressings, fatty meats, biscuits, croissants, fast food, cheese, ice cream, and even nuts. Fat has the most calories and provides the least glucose. Our bodies have no way of converting fat to glucose; we can only do that with carbs or proteins. This is why the ideal diet for Farmers is a low-fat, high-fiber, high-grain diet that includes protein. Whole grains provide a steady source of glucose, and reducing fat helps control calorie intake.

The Farmer's goal is not to eliminate fat entirely. That's not possible, and it's not even desirable. There are some healthy fats that are important, even for Farmers in small amounts. Some fat is essential. In fact, there are a few types of fats that are called "essential" because our bodies need them and we can't make them (very much like vitamins). These essential fats are linoleic acid (an omega-6), alpha-linolenic acid (an omega-3), along with the fish oils EPA and DHA (eicosapentaenoic and docosohexaenoic acid). But that doesn't mean a Farmer needs to eat more fat. Small amounts of these essential fats are enough. The point is that Farmers should reduce fat, not eliminate it. Some good sources of healthy fats are fish, nuts, seeds (in small amounts), and eggs (especially "high omega").

What Should Farmers Eat?

What is the best diet for Farmers? Since they have a tendency for hypoglycemia, they rely on sources of glucose to keep their blood sugar up. Unlike the Hunter, the Farmer needs a steady supply of carbs. The best steady source comes from whole grains, so ready access to a supply of grain is a good strategy.

Farmers have more of an issue coping with fat. High in calories and low in precious glucose, fatty foods have twice the calories of low-fat foods, and it's easy for Farmers to eat too much and gain weight. Fat doesn't provide any glucose, so a Farmer often eats too many calories of fat in an effort to raise his or her blood sugar.

A good example of this is with nuts. A hungry Farmer is likely to overeat nuts, because they have more calories in fat than in carbs. If you snack on nuts trying to raise your blood sugar, it's very easy to get too many calories because of the added fat, and that can make you gain weight. Just a little bit of grain, however, can provide enough glucose for you to feel satisfied. Corn, wheat, rice, barley, oats, millet, quinoa, and amaranth, for example, all fit the Farmer diet: low in fat, high in carbs. Remember that the Farmer diet is low-fat. Eating fats just contributes calories without helping to stabilize and raise blood sugar.

According to the paradigm, the Farmer diet should include anything you could grow in your garden. Staples are corn, wheat, and rice, and rightly so. Those crops can be quickly and easily turned into blood sugar with just a little digestion. Vegetables, legumes, squashes and pumpkins, root crops, fruits and berries, leaves and grasses, and herbs and spices add to the Farmer's palate. This doesn't mean that the Farmer diet is strictly vegetarian. Adding lean protein sources from low-fat sources like fish and poultry are suitable. Eggs are also a good source of complete protein.

Farmers tend to produce more cholesterol; perhaps they've adapted to make more because their diets did not provide adequate amounts. Eating more dietary fat (especially saturated fat) raises cholesterol and LDL levels. So Farmers eating excessive amounts can expect their cholesterol levels to jump even higher.

The Farmer diet is not a license to gorge on carbs, however. While they are needed, too much—especially sugary foods—can cause a delayed blood-sugar dive bomb. Typically that happens when your blood sugar is on a roller coaster, and you're using candy bars or handfuls of gummy bears to rocket out of the lows. Those wild swings in glucose and insulin can make your blood sugar bottom out. That's the classic "reactive hypoglycemia" we see when we do a glucose tolerance test, and the Farmer has low blood sugar after drinking the sweet sugar drink.

Fruit is a good choice for Farmers, even though it provides "fruit sugar," or fructose, rather than glucose. Our body can convert fructose to glucose, but that takes longer, so the sugar from fruits is released more slowly than from a chocolate bar or M&M's. Choose a handful of berries instead of candy, which in addition to some sweetness, also provide a good source of fiber and phytonutrients.

Other fatty foods to avoid are dairy fats found in butter, ice cream, whole milk, and cheese. Nonfat varieties are preferable when possible.

Farmers are best with a grazing pattern of eating. Eating small amounts frequently maintains blood-sugar level and prevents hypoglycemia, so Farmers should always have some sort of grain within reach. At the same time, they need to consciously slow down when they're eating. Just by doing that, normal satiety mechanisms have time to kick in, and blood sugar can be balanced without dive-bombing.

Remember to stick with a low-fat, high-grain meal plan to maintain steady blood sugar and energy throughout an entire day. Here's a table highlighting some of the best choices to include, limit, and eliminate from the Farmer diet:

Best Foods for Farmers	Foods to Limit	Foods to Avoid
Whole grains	Nuts	Fried foods
Vegetables	Nut butters	Butter
Bread	Dark chocolate	Cream
Pasta	Cheese	Sausage
Potatoes	Mayonnaise	Bacon
Cereals	Muffins, scones	Shortening
Eggs	Avocados	Hydrogenated oils
Beans and Legumes	Ice cream	Margarine
Berries	Olive oil	Potato chips
Fruit	Salad dressing	French fries
Seafood, especially fish	Meats	Bologna
Poultry (skinless)	Crackers	Salami

🦋 🦋 🦋

CHAPTER SIX

ADVICE FOR HUNTERS AND FARMERS

The main differences between the Hunter and Farmer diets are the balance of carbohydrate, fat, and protein. Those differences can be easily summarized in the following chart:

	Hunter	Farmer
Fat	HIGH	LOW
Carb	LOW	HIGH
Protein	HIGH	LOW

When applying this type of analysis to specific foods, it becomes clear that some are Hunter foods, while others are strictly Farmer foods, but there are a lot of crossover items that work well in both diets, such as fish, beans, berries, and vegetables.

Fish is an excellent source of protein and omega-3 fats. Small, oily fish are the best choice, since they have better omega-3s and fewer contaminants. Look for salmon, mackerel, herring, anchovies, sardines, and small tuna ("chunk light" varieties are lowest in impurities). The high-protein, high-fat, low-carb profile of fish fits the Hunter profile best, but the "good" omega-3 fats make them suitable for Farmers as well.

Beans are another important food that works well for both diets. Beans are high in fiber, which is a vital nutrient, especially for those who are trying to lose weight. They are low in fat and are generally low-glycemic. By releasing their carbohydrates slowly, they don't spike glucose levels like refined grains do. They also provide protein, which can be a complete protein when mixed with grains or nuts. Choose from a wide variety, including green beans, chili beans, kidney beans, black beans, lentils, peas, garbanzo beans, and soybeans. Their low-fat profile suits the Farmer best, but also provide Hunters with a good source of fiber.

Berries are another food fit for all: Blueberries, strawberries, raspberries, cherries, blackberries, boysenberries, and so on are among nature's best antioxidants. There are even lots of new imported berries like açai berries, goji berries, and maqui. Berries are low in fat and sugar, and high in fiber. The fiber and antioxidant benefits of berries combined with their low-glycemic and low-fat content make them an ideal food for both Hunters and Farmers.

Rich colors indicate more antioxidants, so the deeper and darker the colors, the better. Berries are often sprayed with pesticides, so try to buy organic varieties when possible; frozen organic berries are available year round.

Veggies are suitable for both diets with a couple of caveats. Some of the starchy root vegetables may not be ideal for Hunters in large portions—potatoes, turnips, and other starchy root veggies deliver too much sugar for the Hunter's metabolism. As with berries, the brightly colored veggies provide the best benefits, so it's worth eating a variety of colors—not just greens, but also reds, yellows, oranges, purples, and blues. Veggies also provide some fiber, and they're very low in fat and have little sugar.

How Sugar Affects Hunters and Farmers

It's important to understand how sugar affects Hunters and Farmers differently. Both are efficient absorbers of sugar in all its forms. Enzymes beginning with the *amylase* in saliva begin to break down carbohydrates into sugar before we've even swallowed. Then digestion continues in the stomach and duodenum with the help of gastric and pancreatic enzymes.

Simple sugars like sucrose, lactose, and maltose are released and absorbed by the lining of our small intestine, where they're quickly cleaved for their glucose molecules for immediate energy—blood sugar.

What that means is that a bagel begins to become blood sugar in about five minutes. As digestion and absorption continue, blood sugar continues to rise. That triggers the release of insulin from the beta cells of the pancreas, which lowers blood sugar by causing our muscle and liver to soak up glucose from the bloodstream, and either use it for energy, or store it for later use as a starch called *glycogen.*

But here's where we begin to see some sharp differences between Hunters and Farmers. As we've learned, Hunters produce much more insulin, and it has much less of an effect. The result is that blood-sugar levels are higher overall, and remain higher after a meal. Hunters may still have high blood sugar two hours after eating that bagel. The problem is that when a Hunter eats too many carbohydrates, the pancreas keeps producing more and more insulin as the blood sugar goes higher and higher, which contributes to more insulin resistance, creating a vicious cycle that inevitably ends with diabetes.

So if you give a Hunter a bagel, both blood sugar and insulin climb higher and stay higher than they would for a Farmer.

The best way to bring down that high blood sugar for a Hunter is to move around and do something physical, like go for a walk. Activity helps lower blood sugar by improving glucose uptake by the muscles. Thus, taking a walk after dinner can be the best medicine for Hunters who want to avoid diabetes.

Farmers experience a different response to sugar. Blood-sugar and insulin levels also rise after eating a carbohydrate-rich meal, but much less insulin is secreted by the pancreas, and it works quicker and better, so blood-sugar levels are controlled more quickly in Farmers. The sensitive responsiveness to insulin in Farmers keeps blood sugar lower, and also brings it down faster. That responsiveness can create problems for Farmers, because they'll be more prone to hypoglycemia—low blood sugar.

The pancreas is pretty smart and acts preemptively in controlling blood sugar. It does so by reacting not just to the glucose level in the blood, but also to *how quickly the blood sugar is changing.* If we eat something that quickly spikes our blood sugar because of rapid absorption, say a pack of Twizzlers or a couple of Twinkies, for example, our pancreas cranks out a boatload of insulin because it senses

Of course the results are never too clear. In other studies, salt intake has been associated with higher blood pressure and higher cardiovascular mortality. Increased sodium excretion has also been linked with osteoporosis, because sodium loss in the urine also causes calcium loss.

So the final chapter on the sodium story can't be written yet. No doubt research will soon shed more light on this important topic. But at the moment, we're in a bit of a bind. Low sodium intake is not good, but then neither is high blood pressure. Those able to excrete sodium well and maintain a normal blood pressure are in the best position, regardless of their Hunter or Farmer type.

What about Gluten?

Gluten-free diets are the current rage. They've been touted to be the magic bullet for everything from weight loss to inflammatory and autoimmune diseases—and even your tennis game, according to tennis player Novak Djokovic.

What is gluten? Gluten is a sticky protein found in some grains—primarily wheat, but also barley and rye. It is a particularly allergenic protein for some people and they can become allergic to it. A severe form of gluten allergy is known as celiac disease, which can be a serious health issue that causes bowel and digestive symptoms along with poor nutrient absorption and inflammatory symptoms.

Less severe forms of gluten sensitivity may also contribute to digestive intolerance or milder symptoms such as bloating, gassiness, or fluid retention.

Gluten sensitivity is becoming more widely recognized. It's thought that celiac disease affects about 1 percent of

a rapid and looming influx of glucose that it's going to have to deal with. So it's proactive, trying to stay a step ahead of blood sugar.

The same is true on the way down: When glucose levels are falling, the pancreas quickly cuts its production of insulin. But because a Farmer is sensitive to the effects of small changes in insulin, that commonly produces hypoglycemia. Thus, if you give Farmers a candy bar, they'll like it, but they'll likely be cranky and hypoglycemic in 30 or 40 minutes.

As mentioned, the best remedy is first and foremost to slow down the pace of eating, which slows release of glucose and lowers insulin. Also, by avoiding large quantities of simple carbs, "reactive hypoglycemia" can be avoided. Just a bite or two isn't usually enough to cause problems, but a handful, bowl, or plate full might be.

If you give a Farmer a bagel, he or she should put a slice of lox on it and cut it in half, so that half can be eaten now and the other half in a couple of hours. Remember, Farmers do best with small amounts of carbs at regular intervals.

How Alcohol Affects Hunters and Farmers

Chemically, alcohol (known as ethanol) is very similar to a carbohydrate with one difference: the addition of a hydroxyl or hydrogen and oxygen side chain. Alcohol is converted to acetaldehyde by an enzyme called alcohol dehydrogenase. The acetaldehyde is then quickly converted to acetate, and eventually to carbon dioxide and water. Each gram of alcohol provides seven calories of energy, just less than a gram of fat, which provides nine calories.

Most people think of alcohol as being a source of sugar, but the effect of drinking alcohol is the opposite: it drops blood-sugar levels. Alcohol temporarily spikes insulin levels, which lowers blood sugar. That effect occurs fairly quickly—within ten minutes or so of drinking two ounces of alcohol.

So you can imagine how alcohol might affect Hunters and Farmers differently. Farmers are already prone to hypoglycemia and sensitive to the effects of insulin . . . if you give a Farmer a drink, he or she will be hypoglycemic within ten minutes and will be looking for something to eat!

Hunters are much more resistant to the effects of insulin, and they also have higher blood-sugar levels. So the effects of a drink are much less noticeable in terms of its impact on glucose levels. So if you give a Hunter a drink, he or she will likely be looking for another drink!

You can imagine that the Hunters and Farmers would sort themselves out at a cocktail party: Hunters at the bar, Farmers at the hors d'oeuvres. Of course it's possible for anyone to develop a problem with alcohol, and everyone needs to exercise caution. Sheer calories are among the many reasons it's wise not to drink excessively.

What about Salt?

The news about salt intake might surprise you. We've been told for years that too much salt (sodium) intake is bad for us and will raise our blood pressure and lead to heart attack and stroke. That would seem like bad news, especially for Hunters already at increased risk because of their insulin resistance.

But oddly, studies don't always support the advice to cut back on sodium. Years ago the results of a large national nutritional study NHANES-I involving over 20,000 participants between 1971 and 1975 revealed interesting data. During that time there were almost 4,000 deaths, and those with the lowest sodium intake had the highest death rates, and those with the highest sodium intake the lowest death rate. Subsequent surveys NHANES-II and NHANES-III continue to show the same results.

A recent study of a population of 638 diabetics over ten years found the same results; those with the lowest sodium intake had the highest mortality, compared with the highest sodium intake showing the lowest mortality. Even more recently, results of a study of 3,681 health participants followed over almost eight years showed the same paradoxical results. In these last two studies sodium intake was estimated by measuring urinary sodium excretion with 24-hour urine collections. Those with sodium excretion consistently had higher cardiac mortality. It seems that being able to dump sodium is especially important.

The ability to excrete large amounts of sodium to be protective for cardiovascular disease. Perhaps of that ability is contributing to increased disease.

The name of the condition *diabetes* from the Greek meaning essentially "sweet ancient Greek doctors found the urine of sweet from glucose. It seems we may n of diabetes—"diabetes exsalsus," or uri describe the people more prone to ca Salt excretion may partly explain why be "salt sensitive" while others not so

the population, although gluten sensitivity is more common and may affect up to 10 percent of people. Those with inflammatory conditions may have improvement in some of their symptoms when shifting to a gluten-free diet.

Gluten-free diets are also a new twist on low-carb diets. Since gluten is in wheat, rye, and barley—three common grains—avoiding gluten will also often mean reducing carbs, since those grains would no longer be eaten. It's still not known why some people develop an allergy or sensitivity to gluten. Genetics certainly play a role, and research has identified at least two genes that are present in over 90 percent of individuals with celiac disease.

Nurture plays a role, too, and the timing of the introduction of gluten into an infant's diet may influence the likelihood of gluten sensitivity. One study found that feeding babies wheat-based cereals with gluten at the wrong time increased the likelihood of developing celiac disease later in life. Introducing wheat-based grains before three months of age was shown to increase the likelihood of the disease by a factor of five. That's probably because it takes about three months for the protective lining of the digestive tract to fully form in babies. Breastfeeding may also protect against gluten allergy and celiac disease, because babies benefit from protective antibodies passed on in their mother's milk.

It's not clear whether gluten sensitivity is more common in Farmers than Hunters. Either may have gluten sensitivity if they have the right combination of genetics and exposure. For Hunters, gluten sensitivity shouldn't present much of a problem, since they're better off avoiding gluten-containing grains anyway. For Farmers, gluten sensitivity means having to substitute gluten-free grains like rice, oats, and corn for wheat, barley, and rye.

Gluten sensitivity can be diagnosed with a variety of blood tests, stool tests, and direct examination of the bowel lining with endoscopy and biopsy.

The solution for gluten sensitivity is avoiding gluten, and doing that successfully eliminates any of the potential complications of celiac disease. Even without going through testing for gluten sensitivity, a trial of a gluten-free diet for a few weeks is an easy way to learn if gluten might be causing a problem for you. Most supermarkets today have sections with a wide variety of gluten-free foods.

Supplements for Hunters

Because of the differences in metabolism and predilection for certain disorders, Hunters need to consider different preventive measures than Farmers. Hunters are more often affected by diabetes, high blood pressure, heart disease, stroke, macular degeneration, and peripheral vascular disease.

Hunters tend to produce more oxidative stress—the production of free radicals—which is the result of increased inflammation. Supplements that help reduce inflammation and provide antioxidant support are especially relevant for Hunters.

At the top of the list, perhaps, is DHA, or docosohexaenoic acid; one of the omega-3 oils prevalent in fish. DHA helps lower inflammation and can be protective for the heart and cardiovascular system. DHA usually comes along with its cousin omega-3, EPA (eicosapentaenoic acid), in roughly a 50:50 mix. DHA supplements are usually sourced from fish, but can also be from marine algae. They should be distilled or otherwise purified to remove contaminants.

EPA/DHA capsules are usually in doses between one and three grams per day. Too much fish oil can thin the blood and cause easy bruising. I usually recommend a gram per day, and reserve higher amounts for those who have more inflammation.

Another important supplement for Hunters are probiotics: friendly bacteria that aid digestion and can help reduce inflammation. Probiotic bacteria like acidophilus or bifidobacteria help immune function by replacing unfriendly with friendly bacteria in the gut. I usually recommend high-potency, multistrain probiotic supplements with several types of friendly bacteria and at least a billion per capsule or tablet.

Probiotics work best when taken with fiber, another beneficial supplement. Fiber supplements can be mixed with juice or water to drink as a slurry. Hunters' diets tend to be lower in fiber than Farmers', and fiber helps probiotic bacteria flourish. The best fiber supplements are free of sweeteners or preservatives and contain a mix of both soluble and insoluble fiber.

Another supplement for Hunters to consider is magnesium, an essential mineral found in food sources such as grains, nuts, and greens. Magnesium can become depleted during stress or with excessive sweating. In addition, it can be depleted by consuming too much alcohol, caffeine, and with some medications such as diuretics.

There are different forms of magnesium, but the ones that seem best absorbed and tolerated are magnesium glycinate or chelated magnesium. Others, like magnesium oxide or magnesium citrate, are either not as well absorbed or cause loose stool and diarrhea. I usually recommend 150 to 300 milligrams of magnesium glycinate.

Alpha-lipoic acid is a supplement that helps boost avail-ability of one of our body's most important antioxidants called glutathione. Glutathione is one of the antioxidants our body manufactures to protect us from free-radical damage and oxidation. Lipoic acid is absorbed better than glutathione, itself, and helps protect cells from oxidative damage.

Numerous studies support the use and benefits of al-pha-lipoic acid in diabetes and prevention of complications from diabetes. The usual amount is 250 to 500 milligrams per day.

Hunters have additional needs for antioxidant support, and plant-based antioxidants like lycopene and lutein have shown benefits in protecting cells from damage in macular degeneration and with prostate cancer prevention. Lutein and lycopene are antioxidants found in spinach, kale, egg yolks, and tomatoes. Supplements may help to prevent macular degeneration and prostate cancer.

Chromium is another supplement specific to Hunters. Chromium seems to help improve the action of insulin by enhancing insulin sensitivity. The best form seems to be chromium polynicotinate. Studies in diabetics show im-provements in blood-sugar levels and insulin responsive-ness with chromium supplements up to 500 micrograms per day. The best food source of chromium is brewer's yeast. Lean meats and cheeses also provide some chromi-um, as do black pepper and thyme.

The spice cinnamon can be taken as a supplement, and it has shown some significant benefits in regulating blood sugar in diabetes and prediabetes. Analysis of eight differ-ent studies showed improvements in fasting blood sugar with cinnamon spice or extract.

Co-Q-10, also known as ubiquinone, is involved in energy production in mitochondria in our heart and other muscles and cells. As a supplement, Co-Q-10 may be especially important for those taking statin medications for cholesterol (such as Crestor, Lipitor, or Zocor), as it might help to reduce some of the side effects of those medications. I usually recommend 100 to 500 milligrams per day.

5-HTP (5-hydroxytryptophan) can be helpful for sleep, as it is a precursor to serotonin, like tryptophan. The serotonin boost is especially helpful to the Hunter. This is best given at bedtime in amounts between 100 to 200 milligrams.

Of course there are hundreds of possible different supplements, each with its own purported value, some of which are probably valuable and others probably not. The supplements discussed here have particular positive effects for Hunters, those who are diabetic and prediabetic.

Supplements for Farmers

Farmers have their own weight, metabolic, and health issues. Of less concern for them are the cardiovascular disorders. Farmers are also likely to live a few years longer, statistically, than their Hunter counterparts, largely because of less heart disease. But that also means more diseases of aging like arthritis, osteoporosis, and perhaps even senility and Alzheimer's—and they may be more prone to cancer. Any supplements to help combat the aging process might be especially helpful.

The first supplement in that regard would probably be vitamin D. Long known for its importance for healthy bones, vitamin D is increasingly becoming recognized for its value in cancer prevention and health of the immune system. Studies are ongoing, but the latest research at this time suggests a valuable role for vitamin D in disease prevention. Vitamin D is thought to be more a hormone than a vitamin, because unlike other vitamins, our body can manufacture it when the sun's rays hit our skin.

Ultraviolet B (UVB) rays convert cholesterol in the skin to vitamin D3. A day's worth of sun exposure generates roughly 10,000 IU (international units) of vitamin D. There's a natural mechanism to turn off vitamin D production once enough has been made, to prevent any excess. Maybe in ancient times when we were actually farming perhaps we got 10,000 IU per day but most of us get much less, if any, regular sun exposure. It's worth taking a supplement of vitamin D if you're not getting the sunshine.

Vitamin D is one of the fat-soluble vitamins, so the more fat we have, the more vitamin D we'll need to take. An average-sized person may need up to 2,000 IU a day. Blood tests can be helpful to see if you're getting enough.

Farmers eating the right diet have naturally low levels of saturated (animal) fats, so it's less critical for them to supplement with omega-3's; and their plant-predominant, low-fat diet is naturally higher in omega-3's. Eating fish occasionally suffices the Farmer to provide an adequate balance of omega and saturated fats. Likewise, the naturally higher fiber diet means less need for fiber and probiotic supplements.

For cancer prevention and healthy aging, Farmers may benefit from resveratrol, a plant compound found in grapes and especially in red grapes' skins. Resveratrol is considered a candidate for explaining some of the healthy aging benefits of red wine consumption. The amount of resveratrol in red wine is fairly low, with the highest levels from Cabernet or Spanish reds, which can have up to 10 to 12 milligrams of resveratrol per liter. Resveratrol supplements can be found in a range of doses, but the optimal dose isn't yet known.

Turmeric is a spice used in making Indian dishes, especially curries. It comes from a root that looks like ginger, but it's orange colored. Powdered and dried it becomes a spice, or a supplement. Turmeric contains plant chemicals called curcuminoids that have anti-inflammatory and antioxidant properties. Turmeric is the subject of several clinical trials studying its effects on aging, Alzheimer's, arthritis, and cancer.

DIM (diindolylmethane) is a derivative of broccoli-family foods that has anticancer effects, especially for hormone-sensitive type tumors like breast, prostate, and uterine cancers, but possibly others as well. DIM probably works by enhancing the way our bodies metabolize and process estrogen and other hormones. Typical dosages are 100 to 200 milligrams daily.

L-carnitine is a amino acid–like compound made by our bodies that's responsible for transporting fats into the mitochondria or our cells where they can be burned for fuel. Mitochondria are the nano-sized engines of our cells, where calories are ultimately burned and energy produced. Carnitine helps our body burn fat. It's found in food, but predominantly in meats, so Farmers may need supplements. Smaller amounts are also present in dairy foods. Typical dosages are between 250 to 500 milligrams daily.

The good news is that Farmers should be getting plenty of the nutrients from plants and grains because of their low fat, plant-centered diet.

There are many other supplements that one could take, but these are some of the most worthy of consideration.

There is also the potential for some overlap and crossover in individual cases.

The Hunter's Day

Let's talk about a typical Hunter's day. (This is just one general example—there are lots of ways to tweak the Hunter diet.)

After waking up, the best thing a Hunter can do is to stretch. The Hunter's body type is often accompanied by back pain and muscle tightness in the hamstrings and psoas muscles because of the Hunter's body shape—bigger belly, thinner sinewy legs. It doesn't take much, just a minute or two of stretching the hamstrings, psoas, and quads is a good start.

Breakfast is optional, but a good opportunity to put some fuel in the tank for the rest of the day. Hunger can be the guide, so a hungry Hunter has a few breakfast choices including eggs, cottage cheese, yogurt, breakfast meats (preferably leaner ones or fish), nuts and fruit, a sports bar, or a breakfast bean burrito. Sometimes a protein shake with unsweetened juice or soymilk, berries, yogurt, and protein powder can be a great start to a low-glycemic day.

Small amounts of whole-grain carbs are okay for some, and that might mean small portions of steel-cut oatmeal with berries, or a small slice of high-fiber multigrain toast or unsweetened granola with nuts, raisins, and berries.

Best breakfast beverages are coffee or tea. Coffee should be brewed through an unbleached paper filter to remove the *cafestol,* an alkaloid in coffee that can raise cholesterol. Regular coffee is actually preferred over decaf for Hunters, as caffeine has been shown in some studies to lower the risk of diabetes. Sweetening should be minimal or none: A teaspoon of sugar or less may be better than adding artificial sweeteners in the long run. Adding milk is fine.

Aside from coffee or tea, you might also consider a small glass of pomegranate or other brightly colored, unsweetened fruit juice. A glass of milk or soymilk is fine, too.

This is a good time to take the morning supplements, which would usually include a fish oil capsule, magnesium, alpha-lipoic acid, and Co-Q-10.

Then it's off to work or the usual daily chores. After a good Hunter breakfast, there's usually not much need for snacking or much appetite during the day. If desired, however, a piece of fruit or a handful of nuts and raisins is usually plenty. Hunters will notice that a big meal in the middle of the day, and especially one that is filled with carbs, will sharply slash energy levels and induce a near carb-coma. The less eaten during the day, the more energy Hunters have and the better able they are to perform.

However, it is very important Hunters drink lots of fluids all day. It's better to be preemptive with fluids than to wait until thirst kicks in. Water is best, but tea or coffee are also good choices. Having a water bottle on hand is a good way to improve hydration. Some prefer adding slices of lemon or lime for even better taste to encourage drinking more.

Energy might start to fade later in the afternoon and Hunters can be looking for a pick-me-up. Two ounces of dark chocolate might help—if you can limit it to that. A small glass of colorful juice can also perk you up, as can a handful of nuts or a piece of cheese, some crunchy snap peas, or a bit of hummus.

The early evening is a great time for the Hunter to get some exercise. Jump on the treadmill, ride your bike, go rollerblading, hit the elliptical, go for a swim, or play ball.

Some kind of aerobic exercise in the evening is best for Hunters, especially before dinner.

Aerobic means getting your heart rate up, and that usually means getting it up to 70 percent of your maximum heart rate. Maximum heart rate can be predicted by subtracting your age from 220. A 40-year-old's maximum heart rate should be 180, for instance. Take 70 percent of that (in this case) and you get 126; this is a 40-year-old's target heart rate. The goal is to reach your target heart rate for about 30 to 40 minutes a day. That usually requires some type of strenuous exercise rather just simply walking or most yoga (although some strenuous yoga can certainly be aerobic). By getting that short burst of exercise, the Hunter's glucose and insulin levels are dropped nicely before dinner so that the meal doesn't push levels as high.

Dinner is typically the biggest meal of the Hunter's day and offers the most options. Choose from a variety of protein sources: fish, meats, chicken, turkey, duck, shellfish, or eggs. Greens are a great addition, from salads to green beans, edamame, zucchini, or whatever is in season. Soups like lentil or split pea are a great way to get added fiber and fill up on low-glycemic legumes.

More borderline Hunters can add small amounts of healthy carbs, such as a small sweet potato, a whole-grain roll, or a small portion of wild rice or whole-grain pasta. The key here is to keep portion sizes of these carb sources small. Eating slowly also helps to reduce their impact on blood-sugar levels. This is a good time to take supplements like fish oil, antioxidants, Co-Q-10, chromium, and cinnamon.

Dessert should be considered for special occasions; some options might be berries and yogurt. A scoop of ice cream is actually better than a scoop of sherbet for Hunters, since it has less sugar and more protein. An ounce or two of dark chocolate is another good option. Fruits are fine as well and can be a great way to end a good meal.

After dinner, the Hunter should get up from the table and go for a short walk. This isn't aerobic—it's to aid digestion and facilitate the uptake of nutrients by the muscle and liver. It also helps to control insulin levels after a meal. Just 10 or 15 minutes might be enough, and whatever you can manage will be helpful. If you've got a dog, that's even better —take Fido out for a stroll!

Now it's time to relax. Talk with loved ones or catch up with friends. Something relaxing leading up to bed is best; many people find that this a good time to read, watch TV or a movie, stretch or meditate, or write in a journal. I try to avoid watching the news before bed, which can be upsetting. I prefer comedies or documentaries.

Some Hunters say that the only thing that puts them to sleep is a cookie and milk or a piece of cake, or some other kind of sweet or carb. That's a slippery slope that can become a bad habit. An alternative might be to try taking 5-HTP an hour or so before bed to help boost serotonin relaxation.

A relaxing ritual before bed can be helpful to create a routine that initiates sleep. Some people read in bed, others do some stretching or meditation, and some count sheep. In addition, your bedroom should be conducive to good sleep: cool, dark, and quiet so that you can have the most peaceful, uninterrupted sleep possible. Try to refrain from letting pets on the bed with you because they can unintentionally interrupt your sleep.

If you do need to wake up during the night, try not to flip on the bright lights, as they'll interfere with your pineal gland's melatonin production. Instead, use low baseboard lighting or your phone's flashlight app to allow you to see instead of bright white overhead lighting.

Ideally a good night's sleep allows for plenty of time in both deep and REM (dreaming) sleep, and the Hunter can wake up feeling refreshed and ready to start the next day!

The Farmer's Day

The typical Farmer wakes up hungry and looking for breakfast. It's been a few hours of "fasting" in bed—even though at a very low level of activity—and Farmers nonetheless are likely to look for breakfast first.

Breakfast presents innumerable options from the grains and cereals. Whole-grain toast, cereal with low-fat/nonfat milk or soymilk and berries, steel-cut oatmeal, or even blueberry pancakes or a bran muffin could work. Adding eggs is fine; as mentioned, eggs work well across both diets. Steer clear of breakfast meats, fried or greasy potatoes, and syrupy sweets and doughnuts.

Breakfast beverages could be coffee, tea, milk, juice, or water. (Some people prefer just hot water with lemon.) Coffee, tea, and juices also provide added antioxidants; and richer, more colorful varieties are best.

This is the usual time for Farmers to take any morning supplements like vitamin D, turmeric, DIM and resveratrol, and L-carnitine.

After breakfast is a great time for Farmers to get some exercise. You've gotten your blood-sugar level up, you have plenty of energy, and it's still early enough (hopefully) to get those endorphins going for the day with a quick aerobic workout. Maybe the treadmill, a jog outdoors, or a bike ride. Or consider an elliptical or stair-stepping machine. An early morning workout goes great with the Farmer's physiology.

Farmers should also incorporate some resistance or strength-training exercises into their weekly program. Muscle strengthening, like weight lifting, push-ups, or squats helps Farmers strengthen their bones and prevent osteoporosis.

After your workout you may need a light snack. Remember that Farmers need only a small amount of food to feel recharged and energetic. Now it's off for your day.

You pack along some snacks to keep handy—maybe yogurt, crackers, granola, pretzels, berries, and fruit or veggie juice.

Farmers should stay active during the day. Moving about, standing, and walking even short distances is better than just sitting.

Lunch tends to arrive fairly early. A small lunch is best for Farmers, like a cup of noodle soup and a piece of bread, a peanut butter and jelly sandwich on whole wheat, or an egg-salad or tuna sandwich. Stay clear of fried, fast, and greasy food, as well as heavy meats.

Small portions are best and there's no need to have two courses for lunch. You'll have a snack in an hour or two, so there's no need to eat much now.

As always, it's so important for Farmers to eat more slowly. Eating slowly helps you feel full on less food, as satiety mechanisms have time to send their signals.

An hour or maybe two after lunch you're feeling hungry again. That's a good time for a small snack. Late in the afternoon, as energy levels are fading, is also a good time for some dark chocolate.

If there's a plan to go out to dinner on the late side, it's wise to have a little bite before going out, maybe some cheese and crackers or some almond butter or crackers and hummus. Some might prefer a small salad. Either way, eating a small amount prevents a hypoglycemic gorge on bread or rolls or anything else at dinner.

Farmers may have difficulty when dining out as there are lots of potential traps lurking. Portion sizes in most restaurants are far too big, especially for Farmers who are following a grazing pattern of eating. Chain-restaurant portions are twice as big as necessary in most cases.

Restaurants also add fat to many of the recipes, whether it's butter, oils, or sauces and dressings. Most salads are doused in vegetable oil, which can put even a salad way over the top, fat-wise. Fried or sautéed foods can be too high in fat and should also be avoided.

Likewise, don't order an appetizer, salad, *and* an entrée—that's too much food for a Farmer at one meal. You'll probably find yourself completely full after the appetizer and won't be able to touch your dinner. Chances are you'll need to ask for a doggie bag if you're eating alone, but another option is to bring along a Farmer friend and split an entrée. That way you can even split a healthy dessert and still not have overeaten.

You might even dig into the leftovers at home, later, in front of the TV, and that's fine; or you can save them for lunch the next day, too. Either way achieves your goal to eat smaller portions more often, and to eat more slowly and less. So a small snack later in the evening is fine—perhaps berries, yogurt, a bit of granola, or even cereal and milk. This isn't a meal, though; it's just a few bites. That's how a Farmer can eat low fat and not overeat.

Bedtime may come on the earlier side for a Farmer who's put in a full day that started early. Usually Farmers will sleep through the night and will be ready for breakfast when they wake up the next morning.

Note: Some people will wake up in the middle of the night and, half asleep, forage for food. These people will not remember getting up the next day, but then they'll wonder who rummaged through the kitchen and made a peanut butter sandwich. This unusual night-eating disorder is more common in Farmers who develop hypoglycemia during the night, and then arouse and become semi-conscious enough to go in search of food. The solution might be in providing better slow-release calories at bedtime to prevent hypoglycemia.

❧ ❧ ❧

This is just one general example of a Farmer's day, and there are any number of possible Farmer days and scenarios. The key is keeping from bottoming out blood sugar without overeating. The pattern of eating is also important for the Farmer, who needs more frequent meals and snacks compared with the Hunter.

The varying dietary needs of Farmers and Hunters also means that they are different when it comes to their most common health problems and diseases.

🍃 🍃 🍃

CHAPTER SEVEN

HUNTER/FARMER DISEASES

Anyone can get any disease, and for any one individual, it's impossible to precisely predict what a future disease might be. That said, knowing a person's Hunter/Farmer type can help make predictions about the likelihood of certain diseases. It's certainly helpful for me, as a doctor, because I know what to be concerned about, what to be looking for, and how to help prevent problems in the future.

Hunter Diseases

For example, we know that Hunters are more likely to suffer heart disease than Farmers—as well as other diseases of the circulatory system like stroke and peripheral arterial disease (PAD).

Cardiovascular diseases all share a common thread of *atherosclerosis,* or hardening of the vessels. Atherosclerosis develops as a lifelong progressive accumulation of plaque in the arteries. The rate of accumulation is roughly proportional to the amount of blood flow over time, so direct arteries to the heart and brain along with the aorta and kidneys are especially affected, because they receive the most blood flow. Atherosclerosis shortens life by cutting off circulation to vital organs, and this can be catastrophic as in the case of heart attack, stroke, or aneurysm.

Atherosclerosis has been linked with all of the Hunter characteristics including belly fat, narrow hips, low HDL, elevated triglycerides, and high blood sugar and insulin in both men and women. In addition, atherosclerosis accelerates faster as Hunter traits are accentuated. If a Hunter's belly grows, or triglycerides or blood-sugar levels increase, the pace of atherosclerosis hastens.

Developing high blood pressure can add fuel to the fire, with higher pressures putting more strain on the heart and blood vessels, increasing the plaque accumulation and contributing to a seemingly vicious cycle.

The only solution is for Hunters is to eat a diet that prevents belly fat from accumulating, blood sugar going up, triglycerides rising, and HDL dropping. That's part of the reason why newer drugs like statins and blood-pressure medications have been so successful, because they've helped to slow the progress of atherosclerosis. Thus, medications can help, but they can't help lose belly fat or improve fitness. Without the right diet and exercise, medications are only a stopgap measure.

Unfortunately, the perfect storm of stress, high blood pressure, bad eating, and lack of exercise is the environment where catastrophic things often happen.

Take Justin, for example. For years, Justin, a typical Hunter, knew he wasn't in the greatest shape. He had gained a good deal of weight, and he had been working twice as hard at his job, thanks to the bad economy. Everyone's scrambling, but Justin found himself stretched especially thin and it had been a long time since he'd taken a break; he couldn't remember a weekend he didn't work at least one day. And, he wasn't sleeping well, especially one night when indigestion kept him up. That night he swallowed a handful of Tums from the medicine cabinet, but he still felt queasy and sweaty. So he turned on the air conditioner and vowed to himself that he was going to take a break and take care of himself.

But after a long night of dozing here and there, he woke up in a cold sweat with an even worse pressure in his chest. He knew he had a problem. A quick ambulance ride to the hospital and tests in the emergency room proved Justin was having a heart attack. He was 52.

Thankfully, doctors were able to open the blocked artery and insert a stent to keep it open without any serious damage to his heart. Actually, Justin got three stents: doctors found two other areas of narrowing atherosclerosis that hadn't yet caused a heart attack, but were advanced enough to be future culprits, so two additional stents were put in preventively.

When Justin's blood was tested in the hospital, it wasn't a real surprise: high levels of glucose and triglycerides, low HDL, and high CRP numbers.

The good news is that the experience changed Justin's life forever, and he cut back on work, lost 30 pounds, and became a regular exerciser. He's also taking medications for his blood pressure and cholesterol, as well as aspirin; his blood tests have improved dramatically as a result. Atherosclerosis can be slowed and the catastrophic complications can be delayed significantly with proper treatment.

As I've said many times, Hunters are also much more prone to type 2 diabetes. The combination of diabetes and atherosclerosis is particularly dangerous, increasing the chances of heart attack and stroke.

Farmer Diseases

Farmers are less likely to get cardiovascular disease than Hunters. The predominant features of Farmers are usually protective factors against atherosclerosis—high levels of HDL and low levels of triglycerides, glucose, and CRP. The protection these afford is probably a few extra years of life, relative to today's Hunters, because of less cardiovascular disease.

Current life expectancy in the United States averages 77.7 years, with women averaging 80.2 years, and men 75.1. Farmers may do a little better than average, but their issues are that they contract more of the diseases of aging, like arthritis, cancer, and Alzheimer's. (It's not that Farmers are necessarily more prone to those disorders, but because cancer is the second-biggest killer and Alzheimer's sixth, they're statistically getting relatively more noncardiovascular diseases.)

The chance of a Farmer getting a Farmer disease, or a Hunter getting a Hunter disease, increases as Farmers or Hunters age, or as they gain weight. That happens when they're eating the wrong diet: a Farmer eating like a Hunter or vice versa.

Just as the shape and physical characteristics of both Hunters and Farmers become accentuated when they gain weight, a slim Hunter and a slim Farmer are harder to tell apart. Even their blood results start looking more similar when they start losing weight. And their chances of getting Hunter or Farmer diseases goes down, too. That's the biggest reason for both Hunters and Farmers to maintain a healthy weight—to reduce their chances of getting sick!

A Note on Inflammation

Numerous recent studies have highlighted the importance of inflammation as a pivotal factor in so many chronic diseases, including cardiovascular disease, diabetes, high blood pressure, stroke, kidney disease, and more. Inflammation magnifies the effects of high cholesterol and high blood pressure and greatly increases the risk of heart attack and stroke. Controlling inflammation is an important goal that can help to reduce the risk of these serious events.

New technology now helps us measure even very small changes in the levels of inflammation found in our bloodstream. There are several blood tests for measuring levels of inflammation, including the white blood count and sedimentation rate. Recently, a measure of inflammation called the highly sensitive (hs) C-reactive protein (CRP) became available with even better accuracy and sensitivity than other measures of inflammation.

The CRP test measures the levels of a protein produced by white blood cells in our immune system and by our liver in response to some stress or infection and by our fat cells. Carrying extra fat is one important reason for higher CRP and inflammation. It's one of the main reasons that obesity increases risk of inflammatory and cardiovascular diseases, because obesity increases inflammation.

There are many things that can raise the CRP level including all sorts of infections, injuries, stresses, and autoimmune diseases. Whatever the reason, having an elevated level of inflammation from any cause contributes to cardiovascular and other diseases.

Strategies to lower CRP levels have proved successful in reducing the risk of cardiovascular disease include weight loss, exercise, and some medications (like the "statins"). One effect common to all three is the reduction in inflammation and C-reactive protein. The optimal range for hs-CRP is the very low range below 0.7 milligrams per liter (mg/L). Borderline levels are between 0.7 and 3 mg/L, high levels are above 3 mg/L. Here's a table of target levels for common blood tests:

	Optimal	Borderline Risk	High Risk
Glucose	75–99	100–126	> 127
A1c	< 6.0%	6–7%	> 7.0%
Cholesterol	< 200	200–239	> 240
LDL	< 100	100–159	> 160
HDL	< 60	40–60	< 40
Triglycerides	< 100	100–150	> 150
hs-CRP	< 0.7	0.7–3.0	> 3.0

This is another key difference between Hunters and Farmers. Hunters tend to have higher levels of inflammation as measured by CRP. CRP is even higher depending on the amount of fat, and especially the amount of visceral fat. Visceral fat may be more dangerous because of its contribution to system inflammation.

As Hunters lose weight, and especially as they lose visceral fat, levels of CRP decline and risk drops. That explains why weight loss for Hunters helps improve their health and risks in so many ways. Less weight means less visceral fat and less inflammation.

※ ※ ※

We want our diet to help improve our health. We don't want to lose weight by starving ourselves; that's not healthy. We want to eat the diet that's right for us, and that's a diet that also lowers our risk of disease and helps us feel better with more energy and experience less pain and inflammation. By eating the right diet, Hunters can help to avoid cardiovascular diseases and diabetes, and Farmers can help to avoid cancer, autoimmune diseases, and Alzheimer's.

Of course, it's not enough to know how and what to eat—you have to actually do it! To help you prepare healthful meals, whether you are a Hunter or a Farmer, check out the following great recipes in the next section. You can build on this list of recipes yourself, now that you understand the Hunter/Farmer principles. Bon appétit!

♨ ♨ ♨

CHAPTER EIGHT

RECIPES FOR HUNTERS

In this chapter you'll find some fantastic recipes from Canyon Ranch created specifically for Hunters. Once you understand the Hunter diet principles, you'll be able to experiment and come up with additional delicious meals. Remember to save your best recipes to use over and over again!

HUNTER BREAKFASTS

FRITTATA WITH BELL PEPPERS AND ONIONS

A frittata is basically an open-faced omelet. This recipe is large enough to feed a crowd. Cut the ingredients in half if you have fewer mouths to feed. The frittata is finished in the oven leaving you free to cut up some fruit, make toast, and fill everyone's cup with coffee or tea. Use any combination of vegetables you like, choosing colorful produce in season.

As an alternative to cheddar cheese, sprinkle the frittata with about ¼ cup Parmesan cheese. For a satisfying supper dish, serve slices of frittata with a chunky tomato sauce. Leftovers of this high-protein breakfast entrée are good as a sandwich filling for lunch.

8 eggs

2 cups egg whites

¼ cup 2% milk

½ teaspoon lemon juice

1 cup chopped red onions

½ cup chopped red bell peppers

½ cup chopped yellow bell peppers

⅛ teaspoon olive oil

Pinch of sea salt

Pinch of black pepper

1 cup shredded cheddar cheese

Preheat oven to 375° F.

In a large mixing bowl, whisk together eggs, egg whites, milk, and lemon juice.

Heat olive oil in a large sauté pan over medium-high heat. Sauté onions and bell peppers until tender and season with salt and pepper.

Add cheese and sautéed vegetables to egg mixture, and stir until combined. Pour mixture into a 9-inch cake pan.

Bake frittata in oven until eggs are cooked and cheese is melted, about 20 to 30 minutes. Remove from oven, let cool briefly, and cut into eight pieces.

Makes 8 servings, each containing approximately: 175 calories; 6 g. carbohydrate; 7 g. fat; 219 mg. cholesterol; 20 g. protein; 395 mg. sodium; 1 g. fiber

CHICKEN SAUSAGE

This seasoned chicken mixture is wonderful, as well as flexible. You can make it into patties or sauté it and stir it into scrambled eggs or a quiche. It also freezes well. It is far lower in fat than traditional sausage and even lower than chicken sausage you can buy commercially. It tastes as good as any sausage you'll find. If you are careful not to overcook the patties, they will stay moist. Protein is an important part of breakfast, and this is one flavorful way to get it.

- 1 pound ground chicken breast
- ¼ cup minced yellow onion
- 1½ teaspoons minced garlic
- 1½ teaspoon dried sage
- 1 teaspoon cider vinegar
- ¾ teaspoon salt
- ½ teaspoon ground black pepper

In a medium bowl, combine ground chicken with all other ingredients and mix well. Make patties, using about ⅓ cup of the mixture for each. Place the patties in a large sauté pan. Sauté over medium heat until cooked through, about three to five minutes on each side or until golden brown.

Makes 9 (2-ounce) servings, each containing approximately: 110 calories; 0 g. carbohydrate; 4 g. fat; 46 mg. cholesterol; 14 g. protein; 202 mg. sodium; trace fiber

CHICKEN SAUSAGE BREAKFAST BURRITOS

In the Southwest, breakfast burritos are commonplace: a full meal you can hold in your hand. Add this recipe to your breakfast repertoire, and enjoy it for a casual, yet special morning meal. The eggs and sausage are wonderful sources of protein, and the whole-wheat tortilla, vegetables, and fruit provide a full 6 grams of fiber. Put a bowl of salsa on the table to add some spice. After a while, you may want to design your own breakfast burritos with different types of vegetables and cheese, such as spinach and provolone. This dish also utilizes the previous recipe for chicken sausage.

    4 eggs
    ½ cup fresh broccoli, chopped and steamed
    4 one-ounce low-fat chicken sausage links
    ½ cup shredded cheddar cheese
    4 whole-wheat tortillas, 10" in diameter
    2 cups fresh fruit

In a medium-sized sauté pan over medium heat, brown sausages. Set aside.

Lightly coat the same pan with canola oil spray. Over medium heat, scramble eggs.

Lay tortillas on a flat surface and top with ¼ scrambled egg, ¼ broccoli, 1 sliced sausage, and 2 tablespoons cheese. Fold tortilla burrito-style and serve with ½ cup fresh fruit.

Makes 4 servings, each containing approximately: 380 calories; 42 g. carbohydrate; 15 g. fat; 232 mg. cholesterol; 21 g. protein; 554 mg. sodium; 6 g. fiber

HUNTER LUNCHES

TUNA SALAD

Simple and traditional describes this tuna salad style. Add color and crunch by including diced red and yellow pepper with the celery and pickle relish. Also use canola oil mayonnaise, which is a better choice than the mainstream varieties made with generic vegetable oil or soybean oil.

The safest, healthiest kind of tuna that's lowest in contaminants like mercury and PCBs is actually the "chunk light" tuna, rather than albacore. Smaller fish are packaged as chunk light, and smaller means lower on the food chain and fewer environmental contaminants.

1 can water-packed light tuna, drained, about 6 ounces

2 tablespoons diced red bell pepper

2 tablespoons diced yellow bell pepper

2 tablespoons sweet pickle relish

2 tablespoons diced celery

2 tablespoons canola oil mayonnaise

½ teaspoon Dijon mustard

Pinch salt

Pinch pepper

Combine all ingredients in a medium bowl and mix well.

Makes 4 (2-ounce) servings, each containing approximately: 95 calories; 4 g. carbohydrate; 6 g. fat; 4 mg. cholesterol; 12 g. protein; 246 mg. sodium; trace fiber

SPICY LOBSTER CAESAR SALAD

A Caesar salad is often turned into a whole meal by adding chicken or shrimp, but lobster makes it even more special. A typical Caesar salad would have many times more fat and calories than the Canyon Ranch version here. Our unique dressing has all the flavor of the classic version, but because it substitutes a creamy yogurt mayonnaise base for eggs and oil, the calories are significantly less. If Maine lobster tails are not available, don't hesitate to use spiny lobster from warmer waters. Both are good choices. (Also feel free to substitute chicken or shrimp in this recipe.)

  1 large head romaine lettuce, chopped

  ½ teaspoon paprika

  ½ teaspoon turmeric

  ½ teaspoon chili powder

  ½ teaspoon cumin

  ¼ teaspoon salt

  ¼ teaspoon pepper

  4 medium lobster tails

Yogurt Mayonnaise:

  ¾ cup olive oil

  1 tablespoon dry mustard

  1 tablespoon sugar

  1 teaspoon salt

  ¼ teaspoon Dijon mustard

  3¼ cups yogurt cheese (to make, drain the yogurt in a colander overnight)

Caesar Salad Dressing:

   2 tablespoons minced anchovy

   2 tablespoons minced garlic

   ⅓ cup Worcestershire sauce

   ¼ cup lemon juice

   3 tablespoons Dijon mustard

   ¼ teaspoon black pepper

   2 cups Yogurt Mayonnaise (see recipe)

   ⅔ cup 2% milk

   1 cup grated Parmesan cheese

For the Yogurt Mayonnaise: Combine all ingredients in a large bowl and mix gently by hand until just combined.

For the Caesar dressing: Combine anchovies, garlic, Worcestershire sauce, lemon juice and mustard in a blender container. Puree briefly. Pour into medium bowl and add remaining ingredients by hand until ingredients are just combined. Do not overmix! Pour into jar and store in refrigerator until ready to use.

In a large salad bowl, lightly toss lettuce with ½ cup dressing. Divide into 4 equal portions and arrange on individual large salad plates. Keep chilled.

Increase oven temperature to broil. In a small bowl, combine paprika, turmeric, chili powder, cumin, salt, and pepper. Season lobster tails with spice mixture. Place lobster on baking sheet and place under broiler for 5 to 10 minutes or until lobster is pink. Remove meat from shell and cut into 1" pieces. Top salad with one lobster tail.

Makes 4 servings, each containing approximately: 200 calories; 6 g. carbohydrate; 6 g. fat; 113 mg. cholesterol; 29 g. protein; 620 mg. sodium; 4 g. fiber

ONION AND SWISS CHICKEN BURGER

Using ground chicken made from both white and dark meat will make a burger that is more moist than just using white meat, but the addition of the canola oil to the meat also helps in that regard. When mixing the chicken with the oil and seasonings, have a light hand. Too much mixing can make the meat seem tough after cooking.

This is a fine little burger with the favorite topping of Swiss cheese and grilled red onion. Serve with shoestring potatoes and creamy coleslaw. The bun is optional.

1 pound ground chicken

2 tablespoons canola oil

1 tablespoon onion powder

1 teaspoon garlic powder

1 teaspoon salt

¼ teaspoon liquid smoke

Pinch black pepper

1 large red onion, thinly sliced

5 multigrain hamburger buns

⅔ cup shredded, low-fat Swiss cheese

5 lettuce leaves

1 medium tomato, thinly sliced

In a large bowl, combine ground chicken, canola oil, onion powder, garlic powder, salt, liquid smoke, and black pepper.

Form into 5 patties using a ½-cup measure.

Heat a large sauté pan and lightly coat with olive oil spray. Cook patties over medium heat until cooked through, about 3 to 5 minutes on each side. Remove from pan. Add red onion slices and sauté until tender, about 2 minutes.

Place a chicken burger on bottom half of bun. Top with 2 tablespoons shredded cheese and ¼ cup sautéed red onion. Garnish plate with lettuce and tomato.

Makes 5 chicken burgers, each containing approximately: 410 calories; 44 g. carbohydrate; 11 g. fat; 58 mg. cholesterol; 34 g. protein; 565 mg. sodium; 5 g. fiber

EGG SALAD

Eggs are truly a health food. Their reputation has suffered because of an unnecessary emphasis on the dangers of dietary cholesterol, but they have been exonerated many times over in medical research. They are a good source of protein, biotin, and lutein, a carotenoid that helps protect against macular degeneration. There are many choices of eggs available today. At Canyon Ranch, we recommend organic, free-range, or "omega" eggs. That designation gives you the best chance of buying eggs from hens that have been treated well and fed higher amounts of omega-3's.

Remember, eggs work well for both Hunters and Farmers. Hunters might want to skip the bread and have their egg salad over lettuce or spinach.

7 hard-boiled eggs

3 tablespoons diced celery

1 teaspoon Dijon mustard

¾ teaspoon salt

¼ teaspoon black pepper

⅓ cup canola oil mayonnaise

¼ cup diced red onion

¼ cup sweet relish

3 tablespoons diced red bell pepper

2 teaspoons white distilled vinegar

Chop eggs. Combine with remaining ingredients. Serve ½ cup.

Makes 6 servings, each containing approximately: 195 calories; 5 g. carbohydrate; 12 g. fat; 245 mg. cholesterol; 8 g. protein; 397 mg. sodium; trace fiber

GREEK SALAD WITH RED WINE VINAIGRETTE

This salad is filling and has a balance of fat, protein, carbs, and fiber. This version calls for the tiny, extremely sweet currant tomatoes, but cherry tomatoes or even chopped Roma tomatoes will do. Use whatever is ripe and in season at your favorite farmers' market, produce stand, or natural food supermarket. If you can find organic or unwaxed cucumbers, they can be left unpeeled for a little extra color and fiber.

¼ cup shredded radicchio

1 pound romaine lettuce hearts, cut into bite-sized pieces (about 6 cups)

1 cup currant or cherry tomatoes, cut in half

1 cucumber, peeled and diced

¼ cup chopped kalamata olives

½ cup diced red onion

½ cup Red Wine Vinaigrette (see recipe)

1 cup whole-wheat croutons

½ cup crumbled feta cheese

Combine radicchio and romaine lettuce in a large bowl. Divide into 4 equal portions and place on salad plates. Top each serving with ¼ cup currant tomatoes, ¼ cup diced cucumber, 1 tablespoon olives, and 2 tablespoons diced red onion.

Drizzle 2 tablespoons dressing over salad and toss lightly. Garnish with ¼ cup croutons and 2 tablespoons feta cheese.

Makes 4 servings, each containing approximately: 245 calories; 23 g. carbohydrate; 14 g. fat; 26 mg. cholesterol; 10 g. protein; 624 mg. sodium; 5 g. fiber

Red Wine Vinaigrette:

- ⅔ cup red wine vinegar
- ⅔ cup champagne vinegar
- ½ cup vegetable stock
- 1 tablespoon minced shallots
- 2 tablespoons black pepper
- 4 tablespoons white miso paste
- 1 tablespoon chopped fresh oregano
- 1 tablespoon chopped fresh rosemary

In a blender container, combine all ingredients except for oregano and rosemary and blend until smooth. Add herbs and mix by hand.

Pour into a storage container and refrigerate for up to two weeks.

Makes 16 (2-tablespoon) servings, each containing approximately: 10 calories; 2 g. carbohydrate; trace fat; 0 mg. cholesterol; trace protein; 292 mg. sodium; trace fiber

CEVICHE

Our recipe for ceviche, a marinated fish and shrimp salad, incorporates many Mexican seashore flavors—lime juice, avocado, jalapeño, and cilantro. It is chunky and full of vegetables and color, like Mexican seafood cocktails. Normally, the seafood in ceviche "cooks" in the lime juice over several hours, but we have parboiled the fish and shrimp to speed up the process. Serve this delicious fish and shrimp salad as an appetizer or snack on a warm afternoon or as the main course along with black beans and fresh mango. Use homemade tortilla chips to scoop up the ceviche.

2 quarts water

1 pound white fish

6 ounces shrimp, shelled and deveined

1 small red onion, diced

1¼ cups lime juice

2 medium avocados, diced

¼ cup chopped cilantro

1 large cucumber, peeled and diced

1 tablespoon minced jalapeño pepper

2 medium tomatoes, peeled and diced

1½ cups tomato juice

2 tablespoons tomato puree

1¼ cups clam juice

1 teaspoon salt

1½ teaspoons black pepper

1½ teaspoons sugar

8 corn tortillas, cut into thin strips

Olive oil spray

Bring water to a boil in a large saucepan. Add fish and boil in water for 10 to 20 seconds. Drain water immediately.

Place onions, lime juice, and fish in a large bowl; let sit for 5 minutes. Add avocado, cilantro, cucumber, jalapeños, tomatoes, tomato juice, tomato puree, clam juice, salt, pepper, and sugar. Mix gently. Refrigerate until chilled, about one hour.

Preheat oven to 375° F. Place tortilla strips on a baking sheet. Lightly spray with olive oil. Bake for about 5 to 10 minutes or until crisp. Portion 1½ cups ceviche in a bowl. Divide tortilla strips into 8 equal portions. Top ceviche with 1 portion tortilla strips.

Makes 8 servings, each containing approximately: 230 calories; 27 g. carbohydrate; 6 g. fat; 62 mg. cholesterol; 19 g. protein; 544 mg. sodium; 5 g. fiber

HUNTER DINNERS

PEPPERED CHICKEN MEDALLIONS
WITH MUSHROOMS

The sauce begins its life with a mere ¼ tablespoon of butter but derives its richness, without loads of calories, from our homemade veal demi-glace and 4 teaspoons of heavy cream. If necessary, you can use chicken broth reduced to half its volume instead of the demi-glace. (If you look at our demi-glace recipe, however, you'll see that chicken broth alone just isn't a good substitute.) Properly portioned, this dish is low in calories and highly satisfying because of its protein and fat content. Despite the decadent flavor, it has far fewer calories than a conventional recipe.

Pepper Sauce:

- 1 teaspoon green peppercorns
- 1 tablespoon white wine
- 2 tablespoons minced shallots
- ¼ tablespoon unsalted butter
- 2½ tablespoons dry sherry
- ⅔ cup Veal Demi-Glace (see recipe)
- 2 teaspoons Dijon mustard
- 1 tablespoon plus 1 teaspoon heavy cream

- 4 four-ounce chicken breasts
- 1 teaspoon black pepper

½ teaspoon salt

1 tablespoon olive oil

1 cup fresh cremini mushrooms or seasonal wild mushrooms

1 ⅓ cups chicken stock

Combine peppercorns and wine in a small sauté pan. Bring to a boil and cook until wine has evaporated. Cool peppercorns and coarsely chop in a coffee grinder (use a clean one, especially for spices, to avoid mixing flavors).

In a large sauté pan, melt butter and add shallots. Cook over low heat until slightly browned, add peppercorns and sherry. Simmer for 1 minute.

Add demi-glace and bring to a boil. Reduce heat and whisk in Dijon mustard until combined. Remove from heat and whisk in cream. Set aside.

Cut chicken breasts in half to form 8 (2-ounce) medallions. Season with salt and pepper. Heat olive oil in a large sauté pan and add chicken. Cook over medium heat until golden brown on one side. Turn chicken and add mushrooms. Sauté briefly. Add stock and cook until chicken is completely cooked. Add sauce and cook until heated through.

Serve 2 chicken medallions with ¼ cup sauce.

Makes 4 servings, each containing approximately: 265 calories; 6 g. carbohydrate; 12 g. fat; 79 mg. cholesterol; 30 g. protein; 340 mg. sodium; trace fiber

VEAL DEMI-GLACE

3 pounds assorted veal bones

¾ pound veal leg bone

½ carrot, roughly chopped

1 small onion, roughly chopped

1 celery stock, roughly chopped

1 bouquet garni (see Cook's note at end of recipe)

2 quarts water

¼ cup chopped shallots

2 garlic cloves, chopped

4 tablespoons burgundy wine

2 tablespoons sherry

1½ teaspoons black pepper

¼ teaspoon salt

¾ cup water

1 tablespoon cornstarch

Preheat oven to 350° F.

On a large baking sheet, place veal bones, carrots, onions, and celery. Bake in oven for 20 minutes or until vegetables are roasted.

Place roasted vegetables and bone in a 3 quart stock pot with 2 quarts water and bouquet garni. Bring to a boil. Reduce heat and simmer for 3 to 4 hours, or until liquid measures about 2 cups. Remove bones and bouquet garni and discard. Strain vegetables and reserve liquid (glace de viande).

Spray a large sauté pan with canola oil. Sauté shallots and garlic over medium heat until shallots are translucent. Add burgundy wine and sherry and simmer until liquid is almost evaporated. Add glace de viande and ¾ cup water. Bring to a boil and simmer until demi-glace measures about 2 cups. Combine cornstarch with an equal amount of water and mix to form a paste. Add to demi-glace and simmer about 1 minute, or until thickened.

Makes 16 (2-tablespoon) servings, each containing approximately: 30 calories; 3 g. carbohydrate; 11 mg. cholesterol; 3 g. protein; 47 mg. sodium; trace fiber; trace fat

Cook's note: A *bouquet garni* is a combination of 2 tablespoons each of parsley and black peppercorns and 1 bay leaf, wrapped in an 8-inch square of cheesecloth and tied at the top.

SEARED SCALLOPS WITH
CRANBERRY GINGER VINAIGRETTE

In this recipe, two pounds of scallops serve eight people. That works out to 4 ounces per person, but you'll notice that the recipe says to "serve 3 ounces scallops" for each plate. That is because you can generally count on a loss of about 25 percent weight with cooking. Some protein-rich foods, like seafood, chicken, and meat, will lose less and others will lose more. You should generally count on feeding four people with one pound. For this recipe, you needn't weigh out 3 ounces, but rather portion the 2 pounds evenly among the eight servings.

Cranberry Ginger Vinaigrette:

½ cup frozen cranberries, thawed

½ teaspoon minced ginger root

2 tablespoons diced shallots

⅓ cup apple cider

4 teaspoons sugar

2 teaspoons canola oil

2 teaspoons olive oil

Pinch salt

2 pounds scallops

2 tablespoons olive oil

Combine all ingredients for vinaigrette in a bler
puree until smooth.

In a large sauté pan, sear scallops in olive oil over
golden brown, about 2 to 3 minutes on each side.

Serve 3 ounces scallops with 2 tablespoons cranberry ginger
vinaigrette.

*Makes 8 servings, each containing approximately: 165 calories; 6
g. carbohydrate; 7 g. fat; 37 mg. cholesterol; 19 g. protein; 198 mg.
sodium; trace fiber*

TURKEY MEATLOAF

Here is comfort food at its finest and healthiest. We have made a moist and tasty meatloaf from ground turkey breast. We have added ketchup, egg, and olive oil to keep the meatloaf from becoming dry. But even so, the calorie and fat savings over a similar meatloaf made with ground beef is significant. When you mix the ingredients, handle the mixture gently. If you don't, the meatloaf might be tough. We suggest serving this home-style treat with mashed cauliflower and steamed fresh green beans. A meatloaf sandwich the next day is one of the benefits of making meatloaf at home.

1½ pounds ground turkey breast

1 whole egg

⅔ cup minced onion

⅓ cup minced red bell pepper

½ cup ketchup

2 tablespoons Worcestershire sauce

½ teaspoon chopped, fresh basil

2 tablespoons olive oil

1 teaspoon salt

½ cup Panko bread crumbs

¼ teaspoon black pepper

Preheat oven to 375° F. Lightly coat a 4" x 8" bread pan with canola oil.

Combine all ingredients in a large bowl and mix well. Shape into a loaf and place in pan.

Bake for 45 minutes or until turkey is cooked through. Cool slightly and slice into 6 equal portions.

Makes 6 servings, each containing approximately: 245 calories; 8 g. carbohydrate; 7 g. fat; 147 mg. cholesterol; 36 g. protein; 581 mg. sodium; trace fiber

MASHED CAULIFLOWER

Mashed cauliflower is great whether you're a Hunter or Farmer. It tastes delicious, the texture is pleasing, and it doesn't have the carbs of mashed potatoes. In addition to its low calories, cauliflower is a cruciferous vegetable, related to broccoli, bok choy, and cabbage. As such, it is rich in indoles, a substance that helps the body metabolize hormones and may help decrease risk of breast cancer. Plus, it is high in vitamin C.

- 1 pound cauliflower, chopped
- 1 tablespoon butter
- 1 teaspoon salt
- ¼ teaspoon ground black pepper

In a medium saucepan, combine 1 quart of water and cauliflower. Bring to a boil and cook for 15 to 20 minutes until cauliflower is tender. Turn off heat and drain cauliflower. Add cauliflower back into warm saucepan and let sit for 1 to 2 minutes to dry cauliflower.

Place cauliflower into mixing bowl and add remaining ingredients. Beat with electric mixer until fluffy.

Makes 8 (¼-cup) servings, each containing approximately: 40 calories; 3 g. carbohydrate; 3 g. fat; 8 mg. cholesterol; 1 g. protein; 217 mg. sodium; 1 g. fiber

SPICY HALIBUT WITH HORSERADISH SAUCE

This dish provides robust flavor for those who like some punch. The cooling, sour cream–based horseradish sauce is bold on its own but perfectly complements the peppery rub on the halibut. Try the horseradish sauce on beef tenderloin or even on chicken breast. Serve this with a dark leafy salad and a steamed green vegetable that won't compete with the flavor of the entrée. Wild-caught Pacific halibut is the recommendation from the organization Seafood Watch, as opposed to gillnet-caught Pacific halibut or any type of Atlantic halibut.

Horseradish Sauce:

- 1 cup nonfat sour cream
- 1 tablespoon Grey Poupon mustard
- 1 tablespoon minced garlic
- 1 tablespoon horseradish
- 1 teaspoon black pepper
- ¼ teaspoon sea salt

- 1 teaspoon oregano, dry
- 1 teaspoon cumin seed, powder
- 1 teaspoon onion powder
- 1 teaspoon garlic powder
- 1 teaspoon black pepper
- 1 teaspoon chili powder
- 1 teaspoon sea salt
- 1 pound halibut
- 1 teaspoon olive oil

In a medium bowl combine sour cream, mustard, garlic, horse-radish, pepper, and salt. Mix well and set aside.

In a small bowl, combine oregano, cumin, onion powder, garlic powder, black pepper, chili powder, and salt.

Lightly coat halibut with olive oil and dredge each fillet in the spice mixture. Grill on high heat for about 4 minutes on each side or until done. Serve with ¼ cup of Horseradish Sauce.

Makes 4 servings, each containing approximately: 160 calories; 8 g. carbohydrate; 4 g. fat; 27 mg. cholesterol; 22 g. protein; 593 mg. sodium; trace fiber

🌿 🌿 🌿

CHAPTER NINE

RECIPES FOR FARMERS

In this section you'll find some Canyon Ranch recipes that will make you so happy you're a Farmer. These meals deliver enough whole grains to fuel a day's work. And that starts with the following delicious breakfasts to make you especially glad to be a Farmer! These meals are tailored to be high in nutrients while low in calories, and highly satisfying.

FARMER BREAKFASTS

WHOLE-WHEAT BUTTERMILK PANCAKES WITH FRUIT

This recipe is destined to become a weekend favorite at your house. Celebrate the seasons by adding the freshest fruit you can find to the pancake batter. Blueberries are the classic, but strawberries and raspberries work well also. In the summer, when peaches and apricots are available, try them. Even banana works well. Vary your toppings as well: try jams or preserves with a spoonful of plain yogurt or everyone's favorite, real maple syrup. We blend bread flour and whole-wheat flour for perfect texture. The whole grain paired with the fruit results in pancakes that are a respectable source of fiber.

¾ cup bread flour

¾ cup whole-wheat flour

3 tablespoons sugar

¼ teaspoon salt

2½ teaspoons baking powder

1 teaspoon baking soda

1 tablespoon maple syrup

1 large egg

1 cup buttermilk

¾ cup 2% milk

2½ tablespoons canola oil

1 cup berries or chopped fruit

In a large bowl, combine all dry ingredients. In a medium bowl combine remaining wet ingredients and mix well. Add wet ingredients to dry ingredients and mix until smooth.

Lightly coat a griddle or large sauté pan with canola oil. Place on burner over medium heat until hot. Portion approximately 3 tablespoons batter on griddle and sprinkle with 1 tablespoon berries. Cover berries with 1 additional tablespoon batter and cook until bubbles form. Flip and cook other side to golden brown.

Makes 6 (3-pancake) servings, each containing approximately: 335 calories; 59 g. carbohydrate; 8 g. fat; 48 mg. cholesterol; 8 g. protein; 572 mg. sodium; 4 g. fiber

FRUIT SALAD

As written, this salad uses fruit from a variety of seasons. Please use what is seasonal to make this colorful and nutritious salad, keeping only the simple dressing constant. Even a combination of just two fruits is delicious. The dressing is a puree of orange juice and banana. Thin it with more orange juice to get the consistency you like. The acid in the orange juice helps prevent browning of the fruits prone to that, and the flavor is tremendous.

⅔ cup blueberries, raw

⅔ cup oranges, small segments

¼ cup diced mango

½ banana, sliced

⅔ cup diced, peeled apples

½ cup diced peaches

⅔ cup green grapes

⅔ cup diced pineapple

½ cup quartered strawberries

Dressing:

2 teaspoons orange juice

½ banana

1½ tablespoon diced mango (optional)

In a blender, puree Dressing ingredients. Mix with rest of fruit, arranged as desired.

Makes 10 (½-cup) servings, each containing approximately: 50 calories; trace fat; trace protein; 12 g. carbohydrate; 0 mg. cholesterol; 1 mg. sodium; 2 g. fiber

GRANOLA

This is a wonderful and simple granola recipe that can easily be doubled or tripled if you eat it regularly. The particular blend of dried cranberries and cherries, coconut milk, and maple syrup gives a different flavor than commercial granola. It isn't very sweet, but the flavors are complex. If you don't have cashew butter on hand, substitute peanut or almond butter, or even canola oil. Although granola is whole grain and filled with good fruit and nuts, portions must be controlled because of the nut (fat) content for Farmers.

This recipe is lower calorie than most because it has no oil, but a half-cup serving still provides 200 calories. Portion carefully.

1½ cup rolled oats

½ cup oat flour

¼ cup cashews

½ cup almonds

Pinch cinnamon

Pinch salt

2 tablespoons apple juice concentrate

1 tablespoon pineapple or orange juice concentrate

¼ cup lite coconut milk

1 tablespoon brown sugar

1 tablespoon vanilla extract

¾ teaspoon cashew butter

1 tablespoon maple syrup

¼ cup dried cranberries

¾ cup dried cherries

2 tablespoons honey, heated

Preheat oven to 275° F. Lightly coat a sheet pan with canola oil.

Combine oats, oat flour, nuts, cinnamon, and salt in a medium bowl and mix well. Combine apple juice concentrate, pineapple juice concentrate, coconut milk, brown sugar, vanilla extract, cashew butter, and maple syrup in a small bowl and mix well. Add to dry mixture and mix until ingredients are moist.

Crumble mixture onto sheet pan and bake for 45 minutes to 1 hour, stirring after 25 minutes to allow for even cooking. Remove granola from oven, break apart while still slightly warm and add dried fruit and honey. Cool on sheet pan.

Makes 12 (½-cup) servings, each containing approximately: 200 calories; 32 g. carbohydrate; 6 g. fat; 0 mg. cholesterol; 4 g. protein; 36 mg. sodium; 3 g. fiber

BRAN MUFFINS

In a day when muffins have become as large as little birth-day cakes, these simple bran muffins are a welcome breakfast treat. They are lower in calories and sugar and higher in fiber than most bran muffins you'll find, with 5 grams per muffin. These are sweetened with blackstrap molasses, a nutritional powerhouse in its own right, making these muffins a decent little source of magnesium, potassium, and calcium. Enjoy them fresh from the oven or freeze them after they cool in a ziplock bag. They'll thaw in minutes and are great with a bowl of soup for lunch or a light supper.

1 cup whole-wheat flour

1 teaspoon baking soda

Pinch cream of tartar

¼ teaspoon salt

1½ cups unprocessed wheat bran

2½ tablespoon melted butter

¼ cup blackstrap molasses

1 large egg, lightly beaten

1½ cups buttermilk

½ cup raisins

Preheat oven to 375° F. Lightly coat muffin pans with a small amount of canola oil.

Combine all dry ingredients in a medium bowl and mix well. In a small bowl, combine all other ingredients, except raisins, and mix well.

Add liquid ingredients to dry ingredients and stir just until dry ingredients are moistened. Do not over mix.

Stir in raisins and fill prepared muffin pans ¾ full.

Bake 15 to 20 minutes in preheated oven or until toothpick inserted in center comes out clean.

Makes 12 muffins, each containing approximately: 140 calories; 3 g. fat; 19 mg. cholesterol; 17 g. carbohydrate; 3 g. protein; 240 mg. sodium; 5 g. fiber

BREAKFAST FRUIT CREPES

This is an elegant breakfast entrée for a special occasion. Our delicate crepes are made with whole-wheat flour, and our filling is made with calcium-rich ricotta cheese delicately flavored with cinnamon and lemon zest. Let the crepe batter sit for about 15 minutes before you start cooking. You may need to practice with one or two crepes to get your technique down, but don't give up. They are basically simple to prepare. You can make a batch of crepes and freeze them stacked in between waxed paper to enjoy anytime. This recipe does make a delicious dessert as well.

Crepes:

> 2 eggs
>
> 1½ cups skim milk
>
> ¼ teaspoon salt
>
> 4 tablespoons canola oil
>
> 1 cup whole-wheat flour

Ricotta Cheese Filling:

> 1 cup low-fat ricotta cheese
>
> 3 tablespoons powdered sugar or 2 tablespoons honey
>
> ½ teaspoon cinnamon
>
> 1 teaspoon lemon zest

> 1½ cups fresh blueberries, organic strawberries or blackberries
>
> ¾ cup raspberry coulis (see recipe)

In a medium bowl, beat eggs with wire whip until smooth. Add remaining ingredients and mix well. Mixture should resemble thin pancake batter.

Place 1 teaspoon canola oil in a nonstick crepe pan and heat over medium flame until pan is hot. Pour 3 tablespoons of batter all at once into pan and rotate pan immediate to coat the entire bottom evenly. Cook until edges begin to turn brown and top is firm to the touch. Loosen edges and flip crepe. Cook another 15 to 20 seconds and remove. Repeat for remaining crepes.

Combine all ingredients for ricotta filling in a medium bowl and mix well.

Place 1 crepe on a flat surface. Spread 1 heaping tablespoon ricotta filling in center of crepe. Top with 2 tablespoons berries and roll. Repeat for remaining crepes.

Garnish with 2 tablespoons fruit coulis or garnish with ¼ cup berries.

Makes 6 (2-crepe) servings, each containing approximately: 280 calories; 28 g. carbohydrate; 14 g. fat; 84 mg. cholesterol; 12 g. protein; 155 mg. sodium; 4 g. fiber

Raspberry Coulis:

>1 ½ cup fresh washed raspberries
>
>2 tablespoons fructose
>
>⅜ tablespoon fresh squeezed lemon juice

Puree and strain fruit in a fine sieve.

Add fructose and lemon juice. Mix well and refrigerate until ready to use.

FARMER LUNCHES

JAPANESE STIR-FRY VEGETABLES

At Canyon Ranch, we use our Mongolian BBQ sauce in so many ways, from marinating chicken, meat, and tofu, to dressing a salad. And here it's used for seasoning a vegetable stir-fry. Keep a jar in the refrigerator to use on a whim.

Have all your vegetables sliced and measured before you begin. Stir-frying proceeds so much easier when you can pay attention to your cooking. This is a particularly nutritious combination of vegetables, but it is more of a side dish than an entrée. The snow peas are rich in fiber and the bell peppers in carotenoids and vitamin C. Shiitake mushrooms have anti-tumor and immune-enhancing activity, while the broccoli and Napa cabbage are cruciferous vegetables, rich in indoles that seem to protect against breast cancer.

2 teaspoons canola oil

¾ cup snow peas

¼ cup sliced red onion

¼ cup thinly sliced red and yellow bell peppers

¼ cup sliced shiitake mushrooms

½ cup broccoli florets

½ cup shredded Napa cabbage

½ cup Mongolian BBQ Sauce (see recipe)

Heat wok until hot and add oil. Add vegetables and cook for 30 seconds to 1 minute until vegetables are crisp, but tender.

Add BBQ sauce and toss to coat vegetables.

Makes 4 [½-cup] servings, each containing approximately: 65 calories; 8 g. carbohydrate; 2 g. fat; 0 mg. cholesterol; 2 g. protein; 275 mg. sodium; 2 g. fiber

MONGOLIAN BBQ SAUCE

½ cup low sodium wheat-free tamari sauce

2 tablespoons sugar

¼ cup rice vinegar

1 tablespoon sesame oil

½ cup sake

⅓ cup ketchup

Pinch dried coriander leaves

Pinch dry ginger

¼ teaspoon red chili flakes

¼ cup minced leeks

2 teaspoons minced garlic

2 teaspoons minced fresh ginger

2 tablespoons low sodium wheat-free tamari sauce

In a large saucepan, combine first tamari, sugar, rice vinegar, sesame oil, sake, and ⅓ cup water; and bring to a boil. Add ketchup, coriander leaves, dry ginger, and red chili flakes. Simmer for 10 minutes. Remove from heat.

In a small bowl, combine leeks, garlic, fresh ginger, 2 Tbsp. water, and second tamari sauce. Add to cooked mixture and stir until combined. Store in refrigerator.

Makes 16 (2-tablespoon) servings, each containing approximately: 35 calories; 4 g. carbohydrate; trace fat; 0 mg. cholesterol; trace protein; 288 mg. sodium; trace fiber

YELLOW SPLIT PEA & POTATO SOUP

This version of split pea soup is made with chicken stock with the addition of diced Yukon Gold potatoes and a bit of fennel seed. We love it in the fall and winter when we crave hearty, warm soups, especially in the evening. Dried beans and peas are great sources of fiber, protein, magnesium, and folic acid. Add a slice of whole-grain bread (see recipe) to make a hearty lunch!

1 teaspoon olive oil

½ cup diced yellow onions

¼ cup chopped celery

¼ cup diced carrots

½ teaspoon minced garlic cloves

¼ teaspoon fennel seed

½ teaspoon dried basil

1 dried bay leaf

¼ teaspoon dried thyme

Dash liquid smoke

2 cups diced, peeled Yukon Gold potatoes

½ cup yellow split peas

1 quart chicken stock

1½ teaspoons Worcestershire sauce

1 teaspoon salt

⅛ teaspoon ground black pepper

In a large saucepan, sauté onions, celery, carrots, and garlic in olive oil for 5 minutes or until onions are translucent. Add the fennel seed, basil, bay leaf, thyme, and liquid smoke and cook for 1 minute stirring constantly.

Add the potatoes, split peas, and chicken stock to the pot and bring to a simmer, cooking about 45 minutes or until the split peas and potatoes are soft.

Remove the pot from the heat and add in the Worcestershire sauce, salt, and pepper. Ladle into bowls and serve hot.

Makes 6 [¾-cup] servings, each containing approximately: 130 calories; 23 g. carbohydrate; 1 g. fat; 4 mg. cholesterol; 7 g. protein; 349 mg. sodium; 7 g. fiber

SEVEN-GRAIN BREAD

If you've never made your own bread, it's time to start! Nothing is better than a slice from a fragrant loaf still warm from the oven. You'll find this recipe remarkably easy, and it may become the only bread you use. Look for fresh pecans, sunflower seeds, and ground flax seed; each can become rancid easily. Use bread flour as called for in the recipe. The high gluten content of that flour allows bread to rise and maintain texture. Don't skimp on the salt. It helps the bread to rise.

½ cup pecans, chopped

3 tablespoons sunflower seeds

2 cups warm water (90 to 105°)

1¼ cups whole-wheat flour

1 tablespoon active dry yeast

1½ tablespoons honey

¼ cup ground flax seeds

2 cups bread flour

2 teaspoons salt

½ cup Arrowhead Mills Seven-Grain Cereal

Preheat oven to 350° F. Lightly coat 2 medium bread pans with canola oil.

Spread chopped pecans and sunflower seeds on sheet tray and toast until golden brown, about 5 minutes. Check frequently to prevent burning. Set aside.

In a large bowl, combine water, whole-wheat flour, yeast, honey, and ground flax seed. Let sit in a warm area until doubled in size, about 1 hour.

Add remaining ingredients to yeast mixture and mix well. If using an electric mixer with a dough hook, knead for 3 minutes on medium speed, otherwise knead by hand for 5 minutes. Dough will be elastic but not smooth. Place in a bowl that has been lightly oiled with canola oil. Cover and let proof in a warm area for 1 hour. When doubled in size, punch down and portion into 2 loaves. Place in prepared loaf pans and proof again until doubled in size. Bake for 30 to 40 minutes or until golden brown.

Makes 2 loaves or 32 slices. Each slice contains approximately: 105 calories; 12 g. carbohydrate; 4 g. fat; 0 mg. cholesterol; 6 g. protein; 149 mg. sodium; 2 g. fiber

VEGETARIAN BEAN CHILI

This vegetarian four-bean chili is made from scratch, down to soaking the dried beans overnight and cooking the next day until tender. However, the soaking can be eliminated if you are in a hurry by using high-quality canned beans. We have been recommending more and more that people base their meals on the seasons. This is a cold-weather dish for most people, cooked when bell peppers are not in season. Of course you can find them in the supermarket at any time of year but, next summer, consider buying or harvesting a quantity when they are available at your local farmers' market. Chop them and freeze in plastic bags to use throughout the year.

½ cup garbanzo beans

½ cup navy beans

½ cup black beans

½ cup adzuki beans

Pinch epazote (optional)

1 tablespoon olive oil

1 teaspoon minced garlic

⅔ cup diced red onion

½ cup diced red bell pepper

½ cup diced yellow bell pepper

¾ teaspoon dried basil

Pinch ground cumin

1½ teaspoons chili powder

Pinch chipotle pepper powder

¼ teaspoon dry oregano

Pinch black pepper

2½ cups canned diced tomatoes

3 tablespoons tomato puree

1¾ cup tomato sauce

2 cups vegetable stock

4 teaspoons minced green chili

2 tablespoons chopped cilantro

1 tablespoon chopped parsley

2 teaspoons molasses

½ teaspoon salt

Soak beans overnight. Drain water and add fresh water. Bring to a boil again and add epazote. Reduce heat to simmer and cook for 1½ hours.

In another saucepan, sauté garlic, onion, and peppers in olive oil until tender. Add dry spices and sauté briefly. Add tomato products and vegetable stock, and bring to a simmer. Add cooked beans and bring back to a simmer. Add green chiles and cook for 45 minutes.

Add cilantro, parsley, and molasses and cook for 5 minutes. Season with salt.

Makes 10 (1-cup) servings, each containing approximately: 175 calories; 32 g. carbohydrate; 2 g. fat; 0 mg. cholesterol; 9 g. protein; 189 mg. sodium; 7 g. fiber

BROWN RICE PILAF

This dish is a staple in many households and made even better with brown rice. It's low in fat, and serves up delicious satisfaction that lasts.

1 cup brown rice

1 cup minced onions

½ cup minced carrots

2 cups vegetable stock

2 tablespoons low-sodium soy sauce

½ teaspoon cracked black pepper

1 ¼ teaspoons crushed dried thyme

Rinse and wash rice until water runs clean.

Preheat oven to 450° **F.**

Combine all ingredients in oven-proof casserole dish. Cover and cook in oven for 1 hour.

Remove from oven and serve.

Makes 6 (½ cup) servings, each containing approximately: 145 calories; 30 g. carbohydrate; 3 g. fat; 0 mg. cholesterol; 3 g. protein; 213 mg. sodium

SOUTHWEST ROASTED PEPPER AND AVOCADO SALAD WITH PINEAPPLE VINAIGRETTE

Salads that are assembled on individual plates make quite an impression. This one is particularly pretty with the colorful peppers topped with a bit of mashed avocado and spicy tortilla chips. Stand the tortilla chips upright in the mashed avocado. You can easily roast bell peppers yourself. The best way is to cut them in half lengthwise, seed them, and press them onto an oiled baking sheet skin side up. Roast them at 400° until the skin is a little charred. Cool them in a plastic bag and remove the skin.

Pineapple Vinaigrette:

   ¼ cup frozen pineapple juice concentrate

   3 tablespoons champagne vinegar

   1 tablespoon olive oil

   ¼ teaspoon salt

   Pinch black pepper

   1½ teaspoons chopped mint

Tortilla Chips:

   1 small flour tortilla, about 6 inches in diameter

   Pinch garlic granules

   Pinch chili powder

   Pinch cumin seed

   Pinch salt

🌿 🌿 🌿 🌿 🌿 🌿 🌿 🌿 🌿 🌿 🌿 🌿

   4 ounces organic spinach, thinly sliced, about 2 cups

   4 ounces Romaine lettuce, thinly sliced, about 2 cups

¼ cup thinly sliced red onion

1 small Roma tomato, thinly sliced

½ red bell pepper, roasted and thinly sliced

½ yellow bell pepper, roasted and thinly sliced

½ avocado, mashed

In a blender container, combine all ingredients for pineapple vinaigrette and mix well.

Preheat oven to 350° F. Slice tortilla into 8 bite-sized chips. Place on baking sheet and sprinkle with seasonings. Bake for 3 to 5 minutes or until chips are golden brown.

In a large bowl, combine spinach, romaine lettuce, onion, and tomato. Add pineapple vinaigrette and mix well.

Divide into 4 portions and place on salad plates. Arrange 1 tablespoon each of roasted red and yellow peppers over greens and top with 1 tablespoon mashed avocado. Garnish with 2 tortilla chips.

Makes 4 servings, each containing approximately: 115 calories; 17 g. carbohydrate; 5 g. fat; 0 mg. cholesterol; 3 g. protein; 261 mg. sodium; 3 g. fiber

FARMER DINNERS

Depending on your schedule, needs, and appetite, these dishes might be more than enough for a light dinner, or you may need to combine with another choice or side dish. It's also fine to split portions and eat some now, and save some for later. That fits well with the Farmer's grazing strategy.

CHIPOTLE BLACK BEAN SOUP

A hearty cup of soup can satisfy hunger quickly and for some time. To add a little smoke to your black bean soup, you can add both chipotle peppers, which are smoked jalapeños, and a dash of liquid smoke flavoring. This is a rich black bean soup with a base of chicken stock. Two time-saving strategies include using a high-quality organic chicken stock rather than making your own and using canned black beans rather than starting from scratch. You can substitute two drained cans for the ¾ cup of dried beans in the recipe. Although we suggest serving ¾ cup, a double portion works if this is your entrée.

¾ cup dried black beans

¼ cup diced carrots

½ cup diced yellow onions

¼ cup diced celery

5 cups chicken stock

¼ teaspoon cumin powder

½ bay leaf

⅛ teaspoon dry oregano

¼ cup crushed canned tomatoes

½ teaspoon canned chipotle peppers

¾ teaspoon chopped fresh cilantro

¾ teaspoon salt

1 teaspoon Worcestershire sauce

⅛ teaspoon liquid smoke

2 tablespoons chopped scallions

⅓ cup nonfat sour cream

In a large saucepan, cover black beans with at least 2 cups of water and soak overnight.

Heat a large saucepan over medium-high heat and add carrots, onions, and celery. Sauté until soft, about 5 minutes.

Add the drained and rinsed black beans, chicken stock, spices, tomato products, and chipotle. Bring to a boil and then reduce heat to low, cover and cook until beans are very soft and soup is thickened slightly, about 1 hour.

Add salt, Worcestershire, and liquid smoke. Remove from heat.

Serve ¾ cup soup and garnish each serving with 1 tablespoon sour cream and 1 teaspoon chopped scallions.

Makes 5 (¾-cup) servings, each containing approximately: 140 calories; 24 g. carbohydrate; 1 g. fat; 8 mg. cholesterol; 10 g. protein; 296 mg. sodium; 7 g. fiber

POLENTA WITH ASPARAGUS AND SUNDRIED TOMATOES

1 cup sundried tomatoes

¾ cup 1% milk

¾ water

1½ cup polenta

½ teaspoon Mrs. Dash

Pinch salt

Pinch pepper

2 medium tomatoes

1 tablespoon olive oil

2 tablespoons diced onion

1 pound fresh asparagus

1 tablespoon chopped chives

1 teaspoon chopped parsley

5 tablespoon grated Parmesan cheese

Place sundried tomatoes in a small bowl and cover with hot water. Set aside for about 30 minutes, then drain.

Bring milk and water to a boil and slowly pour in polenta, Mrs. Dash, salt, and pepper. Continue to cook over medium-low heat for 5 to 7 minutes or until polenta is the consistency of Cream of Wheat. Set aside and keep warm.

While polenta is cooking, bring medium pot of water to boil. Cut a shallow x in the bottom of each tomato with a sharp knife. Drop the tomatoes into boiling water for 2 minutes, then transfer briefly to a bowl of ice water. Peel. Repeat boiling process and ice bath if peel is not easily removed. Dice tomatoes and set aside.

In a medium saucepan, heat olive oil and sauté onions until translucent. Stir in diced tomatoes, ¾ of the sundried tomatoes, chives, and parsley. Continue to cook over medium low heat for 10 minutes.

Snap off and discard the tough ends of asparagus. Lay spears in a microwaveable dish with about 3 tablespoons of water. Cover and microwave for approximately 30 seconds, or until they are bright green and slightly tender. Set aside.

Ladle ¼ cup tomato sauce on each plate. Then arrange 4 asparagus spears on top. Add ½ cup polenta at the lower end of the spears. Garnish each plate with 1 tablespoon of Parmesan cheese and remaining sundried tomatoes.

Makes 5 servings, each containing approximately: 330 calories; 59 g. carbohydrate; 8 g. fat; 5 mg. cholesterol; 11 g. protein; 717 mg. sodium

SHRIMP SCAMPI

This is a great Farmer fettuccine recipe and even a little bit goes a long way. The wine sauce is yummy and non-alcoholic wine can also be substituted.

1 pound shrimp, cleaned and deveined

½ tablespoon olive oil

1 tablespoon fresh minced garlic

Wine Sauce:

1 teaspoon olive oil

1 tablespoon fresh minced garlic

1 tablespoon dry oregano

2½ cups white wine

2½ tablespoons cornstarch

¾ cup fish stock (see recipe)

2½ tablespoons chopped fresh parsley

1 teaspoon butter

4 cups cooked fettuccine

In a large sauté pan, briefly sauté shrimp in olive oil and garlic over medium heat for 5 minutes.

In another sauté pan, add olive oil, and garlic. Sauté on medium heat for 1 minute. Add oregano and white wine and bring to a boil. Reduce heat to a simmer and let the sauce reduce by half.

In separate bowl stir together cornstarch and fish stock to form a slurry. Stir slurry into wine sauce and bring to a boil until it thickens. Remove from heat and stir in butter.

Serve 1 cup cooked fettuccine with ½ cup wine sauce and ¼ of cooked shrimp.

Makes 4 servings, each containing approximately: 450 calories; 65 g. carbohydrate; 6 g. fat; 176 mg. cholesterol; 33 g. protein; 308 mg. sodium; 5 g. fiber

FISH STOCK

4 pounds fish bones

3 quarts cold water

1 small onion, roughly chopped

1 medium leek, white only, roughly chopped

4 large white mushrooms, sliced

Juice of ½ lemon

Bunch parsley stems

1 bay leaf

Combine all ingredients in a large stock pot and simmer for 45 to 60 minutes, skimming as it cooks.

Line a strainer or colander with a double thickness of cheese-cloth. Strain stock through cheesecloth. Use immediately or cool and store in refrigerator.

Makes 8 cups, each containing approximately: 10 calories; 3 g. carbohydrate; trace fat; 0 mg. cholesterol; trace protein; 48 mg. sodium

JAPANESE STIR-FRY VEGETABLES
WITH EDAMAME

Stir-fries are fun and easy and deliver phytonutrients and antioxidants. This recipe includes the (optional) Mongolian BBQ sauce (see page 151).

2 teaspoons canola oil

¼ cup chopped red onion

¼ cup thinly sliced red and yellow bell peppers

¾ cup snow peas

½ cup broccoli florets

¼ cup sliced shiitake mushrooms

½ cup shredded Napa cabbage

½ cup shelled edamame

⅓ cup Mongolian BBQ Sauce (see recipe)

1 cup cooked brown rice

Heat wok until hot and add oil. Add vegetables in order they appear and cook for 30 seconds after each addition. Vegetables should be tender, but still a little crisp.

Add sauce and toss to coat vegetables. Serve 1½ cups vegetables over ½ cup brown rice.

Makes 2 (1-cup) servings, each containing approximately: 335 calories; 53 g. carbohydrate; 9 g. fat; 0 mg. cholesterol; 13 g. protein; 615 mg. sodium; 8 g. fiber

PASTA WITH PUTTANESCA SAUCE

Pasta recipes are one of the Farmers' favorites and there are lots to choose from and everyone has their own. But it's certainly easy for Farmers to get fat eating pasta if they eat too fast or too much. Pasta for Farmers is best eaten on small plates, with a very small fork. Here's a great Puttanesca sauce recipe that you can combine with a small serving of pasta to make a great Farmer dinner.

Puttanesca Sauce:

- ¼ cup minced garlic
- ¾ cup diced onion
- ½ cup non-alcoholic red wine
- 2½ cups chopped tomatoes
- 10 Greek olives, pitted and julienned
- 1 teaspoon orange zest
- ¼ teaspoon dried thyme
- 2 tablespoons tomato paste
- 1 tablespoon olive paste
- ¼ teaspoon basil
- 6 tablespoons grated Parmesan cheese, for garnish

Lightly spray a medium skillet with nonstick vegetable coating.

Over medium heat, sauté garlic and onion until translucent.

Deglaze with red wine. Add tomatoes, olives, orange zest, thyme, tomato paste, olive paste, and basil. Cook for 25 minutes or until slightly thickened (the consistency of jarred tomato sauce).

Serve over pasta. Garnish each serving with 1 tablespoon grated Parmesan cheese.

Makes 6 (½ cup) servings, each containing approximately: 70 calories; 9 g. carbohydrate; 3 g. fat; 5 g. cholesterol; 4 g. protein; 110 mg. sodium

❧ ❧ ❧

These recipes provide a few ideas for meals, but there are endless dishes and each could be categorized according to the Hunter/Farmer paradigm.

🦥 🦥 🦥

AFTERWORD

I hope that reading this book has helped you to better understand how different people need different eating strategies and how that helps with both weight and well-being. Eating right is the foundation of good health, and exercise is the foundation of fitness.

Science is beginning to unravel some of the mysteries of metabolism and good health. Discoveries in genetics and life sciences have us looking at things in ways we'd never dreamed. It's likely that we will soon be capable of manipulating health in ways barely envisioned. I hope the day comes when a single pill keeps everyone fit and sound for a lifetime!

Until then, the best plan is to stay healthy and prevent diseases, and that means eating right and exercising. Eating right means eating right for you, and it's probably true of exercise, too. We're learning more about muscle fibers and how they program us for jumping or running distances, for instance, and we're just uncovering how genes might predict musical talent or athletic ability. It is likely that in the not-too-distant future, genes will also be decoded that identify the right diet for the right person.

In the meantime, the Hunter/Farmer paradigm will help you know which diet is best for you, and how to attain optimal health and well-being.

🥢 🥢 🥢

ACKNOWLEDGMENTS

I'd like to thank everyone who has been so helpful and supportive in the writing of this book, especially my wife, Siobhan, who put up with countless hours of my research and clicking away on my laptop. I'd like to thank Jerry Cohen, the CEO of Canyon Ranch, along with Mel and Enid Zuckerman, the visionary founders of Canyon Ranch. They have been intrepid supporters over the years, and their vision and skill has helped hundreds of thousands of people.

I'm especially appreciative of the help and guidance of Christie Hefner, who was instrumental in getting this book off the ground. I also have great admiration and gratitude for Canyon Ranch's Vice Chairman, Dr. Richard Carmona, the 17th Surgeon General, who has been a tremendous supporter and a great champion and leader for prevention and well-being.

Very special thanks to Gene Stone, whom I've worked with on my prior books; I've again found his help to be invaluable. I'd also like to thank Robert Oakes, my research assistant, who has been a tremendous help researching and fact-checking. I'd also like to thank Chrissy Wellington, MS, CNS—one of our top nutritionists at Canyon Ranch—for her expert help with recipes and meal plans.

I'd like to thank my assistant, Kathryn Duffy, and all of the staff at Canyon Ranch who make my job so enjoyable and so much easier.

My editors and publishers at Hay House have been invaluable in helping to improve the quality and value of the book, particularly, Lisa Mitchell—thanks so much.

Many thanks to my colleagues at Canyon Ranch in Lenox, including Dr. Cynthia Geyer, Dr. Nina Molin, and Dr. Tereza Hubkova, all expert M.D.'s skilled in nutrition and integrative medicine. I'm also fortunate to work with our expert staff at Canyon Ranch in Tucson, including Dr. Stephen Brewer (co-author of *The Everest Principle*), Dr. Phil Eichling, Dr. Diane Downing, and Dr. Param Dedhia.

It's a blessing to work at Canyon Ranch, especially with experts like our exercise physiologists, behavioral psychologists, and acupuncturists. May they all continue to do the amazing and healing work they do!

🐦 🐦 🐦

ABOUT THE AUTHOR

A graduate of Phillips Andover Academy and Dartmouth College, **Mark Liponis, M.D.**, earned his doctorate from the University of Massachusetts Medical School in 1984. After medical school he enthusiastically pursued both an internal medicine residency in the Berkshires and Siobhan McNally, an energetic and beautiful pediatrician, who ultimately gave in and agreed to be his wife. They were married in 1987.

Making the "great escape" to the Rocky Mountains, they moved to Butte, Montana, and began their medical practices and their family, with two sons and a daughter born in Butte. Avid skiers and hikers, they thrived living in the mountains, but family ties tugged them back to New England seven years later, and they settled in Lenox, Massachusetts, having come to know the Berkshires during Mark's residency program. That began the next phase of their lives, where fate connected Mark with Canyon Ranch.

Dr. Liponis has been a practicing clinician in internal medicine for 20 years, and also has many years of experience in emergency departments and critical care units. He has always had an interest in holistic approaches to health and began a wellness program as an adjunct to his private practice in Montana in the late '80s. He has continued to expand his understanding and expertise in integrative medicine through his work at Canyon Ranch. He became Corporate Medical Director of Canyon Ranch in 2003, overseeing medical programming at all Canyon Ranch properties.

Dr. Liponis is the co-author of the *New York Times* bestseller *UltraPrevention* and the author of *UltraLongevity*, as well as a contributing editor to *Parade* and *HealthyStyle* magazines. He is a national speaker and has also appeared on a number of national TV segments on health and wellness, including the *Rachael Ray Show,* CNN, the *Today Show, The Jane Pauley Show*, and *The View.*

Dr. Liponis now spends his time writing, leading Canyon Ranch medical initiatives, and striving to be a worthy husband and father to his wife and three wonderful children.

✿ ✿ ✿

NOTES

We hope you enjoyed this Hay House book. If you'd like to receive our online catalog featuring additional information on Hay House books and products, or if you'd like to find out more about the Hay Foundation, please contact:

Hay House, Inc., P.O. Box 5100, Carlsbad, CA 92018-5100
(760) 431-7695 or (800) 654-5126
(760) 431-6948 (fax) or (800) 650-5115 (fax)
www.hayhouse.com® • **www.hayfoundation.org**

❧ ❧ ❧

Published and distributed in Australia by: Hay House Australia Pty. Ltd.,
18/36 Ralph St., Alexandria NSW 2015 • *Phone:* 612-9669-4299
Fax: 612-9669-4144 • www.hayhouse.com.au

Published and distributed in the United Kingdom by: Hay House UK, Ltd.,
292B Kensal Rd., London W10 5BE • *Phone:* 44-20-8962-1230
Fax: 44-20-8962-1239 • www.hayhouse.co.uk

Published and distributed in the Republic of South Africa by:
Hay House SA (Pty), Ltd., P.O. Box 990, Witkoppen 2068
Phone/Fax: 27-11-467-8904 • www.hayhouse.co.za

Published in India by: Hay House Publishers India,
Muskaan Complex, Plot No. 3, B-2, Vasant Kunj, New Delhi 110 070
Phone: 91-11-4176-1620 • *Fax:* 91-11-4176-1630 • www.hayhouse.co.in

Distributed in Canada by: Raincoast, 9050 Shaughnessy St.,
Vancouver, B.C. V6P 6E5 • *Phone:* (604) 323-7100
Fax: (604) 323-2600 • www.raincoast.com

❧ ❧ ❧

Take Your Soul on a Vacation

Visit **www.HealYourLife.com®** to regroup, recharge, and reconnect
with your own magnificence. Featuring blogs, mind-body-spirit news,
and life-changing wisdom from Louise Hay and friends.

Visit **www.HealYourLife.com** today!

a rapid and looming influx of glucose that it's going to have to deal with. So it's proactive, trying to stay a step ahead of blood sugar.

The same is true on the way down: When glucose levels are falling, the pancreas quickly cuts its production of insulin. But because a Farmer is sensitive to the effects of small changes in insulin, that commonly produces hypoglycemia. Thus, if you give Farmers a candy bar, they'll like it, but they'll likely be cranky and hypoglycemic in 30 or 40 minutes.

As mentioned, the best remedy is first and foremost to slow down the pace of eating, which slows release of glucose and lowers insulin. Also, by avoiding large quantities of simple carbs, "reactive hypoglycemia" can be avoided. Just a bite or two isn't usually enough to cause problems, but a handful, bowl, or plate full might be.

If you give a Farmer a bagel, he or she should put a slice of lox on it and cut it in half, so that half can be eaten now and the other half in a couple of hours. Remember, Farmers do best with small amounts of carbs at regular intervals.

How Alcohol Affects Hunters and Farmers

Chemically, alcohol (known as ethanol) is very similar to a carbohydrate with one difference: the addition of a hydroxyl or hydrogen and oxygen side chain. Alcohol is converted to acetaldehyde by an enzyme called alcohol dehydrogenase. The acetaldehyde is then quickly converted to acetate, and eventually to carbon dioxide and water. Each gram of alcohol provides seven calories of energy, just less than a gram of fat, which provides nine calories.

Most people think of alcohol as being a source of sugar, but the effect of drinking alcohol is the opposite: it drops blood-sugar levels. Alcohol temporarily spikes insulin levels, which lowers blood sugar. That effect occurs fairly quickly—within ten minutes or so of drinking two ounces of alcohol.

So you can imagine how alcohol might affect Hunters and Farmers differently. Farmers are already prone to hypoglycemia and sensitive to the effects of insulin . . . if you give a Farmer a drink, he or she will be hypoglycemic within ten minutes and will be looking for something to eat!

Hunters are much more resistant to the effects of insulin, and they also have higher blood-sugar levels. So the effects of a drink are much less noticeable in terms of its impact on glucose levels. So if you give a Hunter a drink, he or she will likely be looking for another drink!

You can imagine that the Hunters and Farmers would sort themselves out at a cocktail party: Hunters at the bar, Farmers at the hors d'oeuvres. Of course it's possible for anyone to develop a problem with alcohol, and everyone needs to exercise caution. Sheer calories are among the many reasons it's wise not to drink excessively.

What about Salt?

The news about salt intake might surprise you. We've been told for years that too much salt (sodium) intake is bad for us and will raise our blood pressure and lead to heart attack and stroke. That would seem like bad news, especially for Hunters already at increased risk because of their insulin resistance.

But oddly, studies don't always support the advice to cut back on sodium. Years ago the results of a large national nutritional study NHANES-I involving over 20,000 participants between 1971 and 1975 revealed interesting data. During that time there were almost 4,000 deaths, and those with the lowest sodium intake had the highest death rates, and those with the highest sodium intake the lowest death rate. Subsequent surveys NHANES-II and NHANES-III continue to show the same results.

A recent study of a population of 638 diabetics over ten years found the same results; those with the lowest sodium intake had the highest mortality, compared with the highest sodium intake showing the lowest mortality. Even more recently, results of a study of 3,681 healthy participants followed over almost eight years showed the same paradoxical results. In these last two studies, sodium intake was estimated by measuring urinary sodium excretion with 24-hour urine collections. Those with low sodium excretion consistently had higher cardiovascular mortality. It seems that being able to dump sodium is especially important.

The ability to excrete large amounts of sodium seems to be protective for cardiovascular disease. Perhaps the lack of that ability is contributing to increased cardiovascular disease.

The name of the condition *diabetes mellitus* comes from the Greek meaning essentially "sweet urine," because ancient Greek doctors found the urine of diabetics to be sweet from glucose. It seems we may need another form of diabetes—"diabetes exsalsus," or urine without salt—to describe the people more prone to cardiovascular disease. Salt excretion may partly explain why some people might be "salt sensitive" while others not so much.

Of course the results are never too clear. In other studies, salt intake has been associated with higher blood pressure and higher cardiovascular mortality. Increased sodium excretion has also been linked with osteoporosis, because sodium loss in the urine also causes calcium loss.

So the final chapter on the sodium story can't be written yet. No doubt research will soon shed more light on this important topic. But at the moment, we're in a bit of a bind. Low sodium intake is not good, but then neither is high blood pressure. Those able to excrete sodium well and maintain a normal blood pressure are in the best position, regardless of their Hunter or Farmer type.

What about Gluten?

Gluten-free diets are the current rage. They've been touted to be the magic bullet for everything from weight loss to inflammatory and autoimmune diseases—and even your tennis game, according to tennis player Novak Djokovic.

What is gluten? Gluten is a sticky protein found in some grains—primarily wheat, but also barley and rye. It is a particularly allergenic protein for some people and they can become allergic to it. A severe form of gluten allergy is known as celiac disease, which can be a serious health issue that causes bowel and digestive symptoms along with poor nutrient absorption and inflammatory symptoms.

Less severe forms of gluten sensitivity may also contribute to digestive intolerance or milder symptoms such as bloating, gassiness, or fluid retention.

Gluten sensitivity is becoming more widely recognized. It's thought that celiac disease affects about 1 percent of

Those sources of carbs are quickly turned into glucose and spike blood glucose and insulin levels. This is especially true of the refined or "white" grains including white flour, white rice, white pasta, and so on.

If you've been a habitual user of sugar, sweets, and carbs for their mood-boosting effects and you plan to break the habit, you ought to prepare as best you can. You'll need to boost your own serotonin levels as much as possible. In addition to exercise, it's also important to maintain a healthy vitamin D level. Be sure to get some sun exposure (no sunburns, please!) or take a vitamin D supplement. Most people could benefit from taking 2,000 IU of vitamin D3 daily, unless you get regular sun exposure.

The amino acid tryptophan is a precursor for serotonin synthesis, so it's important to have enough tryptophan on board. Meats are good sources; you've probably heard of the "turkey-dinner effect," because turkey is a good source of tryptophan. It's also available in supplements in the form of 5-HTP, which is sometimes recommended for help with mood or sleep.

Physical touch can help, too. Intimacy and sexuality boost serotonin and other feel-good hormones. Massage is an excellent way to lessen some of the pain of going through carb withdrawal. Acupuncture can also play a tremendous role in stimulating the relaxation response and positive energy flow.

Dark chocolate seems to benefit some people, but for many, it's very difficult to eat just a little. In fact, sometimes it's better not to start at all, unless you can truly limit portion size. Chocolate can become another addiction.

Withdrawal is a sort of agitated discomfort, so anything that calms the nerves is helpful. Try herbal teas, hot tubs, candles and aromas, massages and body treatments, all of which can help soften the edge of carbohydrate withdrawal.

Some people prefer to go cold turkey and suffer all of the withdrawal, agitation, and cravings at once, rather than stretching out the misery for days or weeks. In my practice I have noticed that it takes two to three weeks for most people to cut their carbohydrate addiction if they follow the cold-turkey route. The good news is that once you've successfully cut out quick carbs, the craving for them goes down, so it's easier to stay away from them once they're out of your system.

※ ※ ※

Not every Hunter needs to eliminate carbs—some just need to reduce. This depends on how severe the effects are and how your blood tests look. Hunters should always consider the *quantity* of carbs. Portion size is key. I'd worry less about a teaspoon of sugar in a cup of coffee, which is only about 20 calories, compared with a plate of pasta or a piece of pie, which can be hundreds.

One simple way to know the quantity of carbs is by counting up the calories in whatever you're eating. Carbs provide 4 calories per gram, or about 113 calories per ounce. For alcohol, figure on 7 carb calories per gram of alcohol for pure alcohol, or about half that for 100 proof vodka, for example. A 1.5-ounce shot of 70-proof vodka would contain about 85 calories. Wine provides around 20 calories per ounce. A typical 5-ounce glass of red or white wine is about 100 calories of carbs.

A slice of bread, depending on the size and its ingredients, would usually have between 20 and 40 grams of carbs, or about 80 to 160 calories of carbs per slice. A plate of pasta at a restaurant can contain as much as 600 to 800 calories of carbs.

Becoming carb savvy is an important skill for the Hunter. It's wise to know how many carbs are in common foods and dishes, as that will help you make the best choices in any situation.

By the way, the biggest benefit to Hunters in cutting back on carbs is the immediate improvement in energy. It's often not until you get off the carbs that you realize how much they were negatively affecting your energy and disposition.

What Should Hunters Eat?

So what is the best diet for a Hunter? Since you know that the main trait of the Hunter is high blood sugar, then the ideal diet should be low in sugar and sources of blood sugar (like grains). The Hunter diet is, after all, a low-carbohydrate diet.

That doesn't mean this is a carnivore or all-meat diet. It just means that while Hunters have carbohydrate intolerance, they are relatively better at handling fat and protein. The ideal diet would be similar to what our ancestors consumed: an actual hunting-and-gathering diet that included game but also fruits, nuts, roots, bugs, fish, birds, and leaves.

What wasn't part of our primary ancestral hunter-gatherer diet were grains and their derivatives; those entered the human diet roughly 13,000 years ago. Grains and their derivatives are among the highest carbohydrate foods. Concentrated forms of grains include high-fructose corn syrup and alcohol, which are particularly difficult for

Hunters' metabolism to deal with. The quicker any food is converted to sugar, the worse it is for Hunters in any quantity. Thus, milled grains like cereals, white flour, white rice, and refined grains of all kinds are the biggest offenders, since they're converted more quickly to pure sugar, namely *glucose.* The bottom line is that large portions of refined and "white" grains should be minimized, if not eliminated, in the Hunter's diet.

Likewise, sweets and sugary foods are especially damaging, requiring very little digestion for immediate conversion to glucose. Large portions can spike a Hunter's blood sugar for several hours. Prolonged high blood sugar begins to cause microscopic damage to the blood vessels, the eyes, nerve endings, and so forth, accelerating the progress to diabetes.

Hunters need some intake of glucose, of course. Without a regular supply, our bodies will use protein sources and convert those to glucose. Hunters' glucose sources should provide a slow, steady release into the bloodstream, so low-glycemic foods are ideal. Beans and berries, for example, are a low-glycemic source of glucose that won't spike blood-sugar levels. Likewise, most vegetables also provide low-glycemic sources of glucose; the sugar content of vegetables is low and released slowly without spiking blood sugar. Beans and berries are high in fiber, which helps to slow their release of glucose while providing us the added benefits of more fiber.

Most fruits are sweeter and capable of delivering too much sugar, especially when it's concentrated as in fruit juice or dried fruits. The good news is that fruit sugar (fructose) requires conversion to glucose to produce blood sugar; so eating fruit is actually low glycemic. However, that's only true in small quantities, as with eating fruit,